The hands-on guide to imaging

D1055723

Dedications

To my parents, Kenneth and Margaret and also my children, Thomas and Ella.
David Howlett

To Janet and Jenny.
Brian Ayers

The hands-on guide to imaging

DAVID C. HOWLETT
MRCP, FRCR

BRIAN AYERS
MD, FRCR

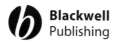

Blackwell
Publishing

© 2004 D.C. Howlett and A.B. Ayers
Published by Blackwell Publishing Ltd
Blackwell Publishing, Inc., 350 Main Street, Malden, Massachusetts 02148-5020, USA
Blackwell Publishing Ltd, 9600 Garsington Road, Oxford OX4 2DQ, UK
Blackwell Publishing Asia Pty Ltd, 550 Swanston Street, Carlton, Victoria 3053, Australia

First published 2004

Library of Congress Cataloging-in-Publication Data
Howlett, David C.
    The hands-on guide to imaging / David C. Howlett, Brian Ayers.
        p. ; cm.
    Includes bibliographical references and index.
    ISBN 1-4051-1551-3
    1. Diagnostic imaging—Handbooks, manuals, etc.
    [DNLM: 1. Diagnostic Imaging—methods—Handbooks.   WN 39 H864h
2004] I. Ayers, Brian, MD. II. Title.
    RC78.7.D53H69   2004
    616.07′57—dc22   2004010888

A catalogue record for this title is available from the British Library

Set in 8/9.5 Erhardt by SNP Best-set Typesetter Ltd., Hong Kong
Printed and bound in the United Kingdom by MPG Books Ltd, Bodmin

Commissioning Editor: Vicki Noyes
Development Editor: Geraldine Jeffers
Editorial Assistant: Nic Ulyatt
Production Controller: Kate Charman

For further information on Blackwell Publishing, visit our website:
http://www.blackwellpublishing.com

Contents

List of contributors

A.T. Ahuja MBBS(Bom) MD(Bom) FRCR FHKCR FHKAM(Radiology), Professor, Department of Diagnostic Radiology, Prince of Wales Hospital, Hong Kong

F. Alyas MRCP, Specialist Registrar, Radiology, Guy's & St Thomas' NHS Trust

A.B. Ayers MD FRCR, Consultant Radiologist, Guy's & St Thomas' NHS Trust

D.C. Howlett MRCP FRCR, Consultant Radiologist, East Sussex Hospitals NHS Trust, Eastbourne

D.V. Hughes MRCP FRCR, Consultant Radiologist, East Sussex Hospitals NHS Trust, Eastbourne

E. Ruffell FRCP FRCR, Consultant Radiologist, East Sussex Hospitals NHS Trust, Eastbourne

D.F. Sallomi DMRD FRCR, Consultant Radiologist, East Sussex Hospitals NHS Trust, Eastbourne

G.M.T. Watson MRCP FRCR, Consultant Radiologist, East Sussex Hospitals NHS Trust, Eastbourne

E.H.Y. Yuen MBChB(CUHK) FRCR FHKCR FHKAM(Radiology), Senior Medical Officer, Department of Radiology, Prince of Wales Hospital, Hong Kong

Foreword

I am very pleased indeed to write this foreword and to welcome the Hands on Guide to Imaging. The authors in their preface have correctly diagnosed two problems for preregistration house officers (PRHO's) and other junior doctors working at the boundary of direct clinical care for patients and radiological investigation. The first problem is the relative lack of exposure in the undergraduate curriculum to radiological practice—there may be plenty of gazing at X-rays, CT scans, ultrasounds etc, but not enough attention paid to how to get to this end result. The second problem is the paradox in the PRHO's role between still being in effect a student or trainee at a very early stage on a very new and steep learning curve yet still needing to make important and executive decisions. This paradox is ideally resolved by junior colleagues having guidance, advice, support from senior colleagues and access to very practical guidebooks written by experienced practitioners. This is just such a book which will guide junior doctors clearly through the practicalities of how to start and then continue the radiological investigation of a patient and what to look for when interpreting the image. Not only will it serve the trainee well, but also patients, and if medical students pick it up and are stimulated to delve deeper into radiology then that will be a well deserved bonus for the authors and editors.

D. Gwyn Williams
Dean,
Guy's, King's and St. Thomas' School
of Medicine

Preface

The authors, as busy practicing radiologists, have had long experience of seeing junior doctors juggle the tasks of the day-to-day management of patients in hospital. As the most junior members of the medical team, they are often expected to have the capability of managing everyday arrangements for investigations, referrals and treatment. It can be challenging when seniors expect newly qualified doctors to have adequate experience.

Clinical radiology is not seen as a mainstream subject in the undergraduate curriculum, and medical schools vary in the amount of training that they provide for their students in the subject. The knowledge that medical students gain is often obtained through clinicians, not through radiologists. This book has been written to fill that gap. It is not designed to be a textbook of radiology, but has been laid out to provide pragmatic advice regarding imaging services specifically for senior medical students and house officers. Rapid advances in imaging have added to the complexities.

The contents of the book have been chosen following a survey identifying the preferences of a group of senior medical students and junior house officers.

Quite understandably, the text of a 'hands-on guide' gives only a limited amount of specialized knowledge and referral to the larger textbooks of radiology is necessary in many circumstances when an in-depth knowledge is required. What we hope the reader will gain is practical knowledge of how to obtain the best service from the imaging departments, how to interpret some of the basic findings and how to avoid falling into the many pitfalls that are waiting for them.

This book will not receive any awards for literary style. We do not apologize, for we recognize that time is short in the busy day of a house officer and that messages have to be conveyed quickly. We have specified what is covered at the beginning of each chapter to assist with easy access, and used bullet points widely to get over the essential features at a glance.

We have tried to make it fun, so please enjoy and learn at the same time.

Brian Ayers & David Howlett

Acknowledgements

The editors would like to thank Louise Pellett for typing of the manuscript, Nick Taylor for preparation of the illustrations and also their radiological colleagues, Nigel Marchbank and Hugh Anderson for access to their film collections.

Abbreviations

A&E	accident and emergency department	IUCD	intrauterine contraceptive device
AP	anterior posterior	IV	intravenous
AV	arteriovenous	IVU	intravenous urogram
AXR	abdominal X-ray	MDP	methylene diphosphonate
BIF	bifurcation	MEN	multiple endocrine neoplasia
COPD	chronic obstructive pulmonary disease	MR	magnetic resonance
		MRA	magnetic resonance angiography
CRP	C-reactive protein		
CSF	cerebrospinal fluid	MRCP	magnetic resonance cholangiopancreatography
CT	computed tomography		
CTAP	CT angiography and portography	MRI	magnetic resonance imaging
		MRSA	methicillin resistant *Staphylococcus aureus*
CTR	cardiothoracic ratio		
CVA	cerebrovascular accident	MS	multiple sclerosis
CXR	chest X-ray	NBM	nil by mouth
DCIS	ductal carcinoma *in situ*	NICE	National Institute for Clinical Excellence
DEXA	dual X-ray absorptiometry		
DVT	deep venous thrombosis	NM	nuclear medicine
ECA	external carotid artery	PA	posteroanterior
EDH	extradural haematoma	PACS	picture archiving and communication system
ERCP	endoscopic retrograde cholangiopancreatography		
		PE	pulmonary embolus/embolism
ESR	erythrocyte sedimentation rate		
		PET	positron emission tomography
FDG	flurodeoxyglucose		
FLAIR	fluid attenuated inversion recovery sequence	PSA	prostate-specific antigen
		PTC	percutaneous transhepatic cholangiography
FNAC	fine needle aspiration cytology		
		PUJ	pelviureteric junction
GCS	Glasgow coma score	rtPA	recombinant tissue plasminogen activator
GI	gastrointestinal		
HRCT	high-resolution CT	SAH	subarachnoid haemorrhage
ICA	internal carotid artery	SDH	subdural haematoma
IRMER	ionizing radiation (medical exposure) regulations	STIR	short term inversion recovery
		SVC	superior vena cava

SVCO	superior vena cava obstruction	TIA	transient ischaemic attack
TB	tuberculosis	TSH	thyroid-stimulating hormone
^{99m}Tc	technetium-99m	US	ultrasound
TCC	transitional cell carcinoma	V/Q	ventilation–perfusion

Chapter 1: **Making the best use of the radiology department**

This chapter covers:
- Historical perspective
- Guidelines and protocols
- Radiation doses
- Patient safety
- Informed consent
- Using the imaging department

Historical perspective

On 8 November 1895 Roentgen discovered the new phenomenon of X-rays. On 3 February 1896 the first of many lecture demonstrations, which were popular at the time, took place at St Thomas' Hospital, London. A student's hand was examined using a 6-inch coil and 24-volt accumulators. By October of the same year, the hospital had introduced a clinical service. This was repeated concurrently across the UK. The take up was rapid and exponential.

Exposure times for radiographs were in the range of 15–30 minutes. There was frantic activity and new designs for tubes and tables abounded. At the same time, Edison discovered the calcium tungstate screen for recording the image, allowing shorter exposure times.

Unfortunately, the harmful adverse effects of irradiation were not recognized immediately and many pioneers received large doses in the first few months until radiation dermatitis and conjunctivitis were recognized and described. Over the next few months and years, more serious conditions came to light that were related to prolonged exposure (e.g. aplastic anaemia). By 1905, X-ray workers had begun to take measures to protect themselves, but for many it was too late and some died.

Rules and legislation were introduced to control the use of ionizing radiation in medical diagnosis and treatment but the first real code of practice, which included protective lead aprons and screens, was not accepted until 1915. It was claimed that commercial interests were delaying the development of proper protection measures.

The most recent set of such regulations are the ionizing radiation (medical exposure) regulations (IRMER) 2000, which are legally binding. These place a burden of responsibility on all those involved in the use of ionizing radiation in patient management. Until a few years ago, the regulations were mainly directed at those individuals providing the service, but the most recent regulations also emphasize the need for those referring patients for examinations to understand the basis of the adverse effects of ionizing radiation and to ensure that on balance the patient benefits outweigh the risks.

First of all do no harm is still a very important principle.

Although more recent scientific developments have introduced imaging modalities that do not involve ionizing radiation and are less harmful, there is a need to continue such vigilance so that no harm comes to patients. All imaging techniques use some form of energy and

1

have the potential to cause harm if things go wrong. This is the main justification for having centralized departments of imaging rather than allowing instruments and machines to be disbursed widely across hospitals or in the community.

The second important reason is one of efficiency. Modern imaging equipment is very expensive and the highly skilled staff who use it have to be well trained. This is a limited resource and careful management is important.

The third reason is that, over the last decade or so, imaging has changed dramatically and it is only the specialists in the field who can manage to keep up to date and to be fully informed of the new developments from which patients can benefit. At the same time, there have been considerable developments within the clinical fields so that treatment options are considerably more extensive and it is difficult for the radiologist to keep up too.

In practice, the patient benefits most when the skills and knowledge of both the clinician and radiologist work in harmony. As you read this book you will recognize this is a constant theme. Communication between the clinical team and the imaging/radiology departments is absolutely essential to avoid harm to patients and to get the very best results for them.

Guidelines and protocols

As medicine has become more and more complex it has been deemed fit to develop guidelines and protocols to help guide decision making as to which investigation is the correct one to be under-

taken within any clinical situation. The Royal College of Radiologists has developed guidelines and protocols for a wide range of common clinical situations and has published these in booklet form (*Making the Best Use of a Department of Clinical Radiology*).

The guidelines emphasize that every investigation should be considered carefully to ensure that it is useful — that it will change management or, at the very least, lead to significant improvement in the confidence of the clinician in the patient's diagnosis.

In many circumstances this does not seem to be fulfilled. To junior doctors this can be a confusing and stressful area of practice. To help you there are some basic questions that you can ask yourself whenever you believe that you should refer a patient for imaging.

• *Has it been done already?* The evidence is that too many tests are repeated unnecessarily when a little effort to find the previous results will suffice.

• *Does the patient need it?* Will the patient benefit from the result and if so how?

• *When is the best time to perform the investigation?* There is considerable pressure and indeed an expectation for immediacy, but this is not always best for the patient. In many circumstances better results are obtained after the acute event has subsided, when investigation parameters can be optimized. A good opinion cannot be obtained from poor images! So-called 'routine' supine chest X-ray (CXR) on admission through the accident and emergency department (A&E) is an example.

• *Is this test the best one?* The range of possibilities is often wide. As a young doctor, you cannot be expected to know about or understand them all. The guidelines will help in common situations but otherwise you will need advice—ask the radiologist.

• *Is the problem and the question to be answered clear?* The radiologist needs to understand these so that the right examination can be undertaken. The wrong test will give the wrong result and not benefit the patient. If you are not sure, discuss it with the radiologist.

Radiation doses

To give you some idea of the range of radiation doses that radiological investigations entail, Table 1.1 lists a few.

Background irradiation varies, but another way of looking at this is to remember that the dose received from a modern CXR is equivalent to the extra radiation received during a couple of flights to Majorca!

Patient safety

Radiation is not the only risk to patient safety in an imaging department. Others that you should be aware of include the following.

Identification

Unfortunately, identification errors abound in practice. Fortunately, few lead to actual harm but some do. Identification errors occur at any point in the process from request to report transmission to the patient. The responsibility starts with the referring clinician to ensure that the patient's personal information provided is accurate. Further responsibility lies with the radiology department and its staff—the radiographers, radiologists, clerks, typists and administrators—to ensure that the films or images and the report are allocated correctly to a single patient.

Misidentification is the most common cause for failure to find previous examinations, and this leads to delay and to unnecessary repeats. One hopes that computerization of patient records will help to overcome this problem in the future.

Iodine hypersensitivity

Many X-ray contrast agents contain iodine and there is a known incidence of hypersensitivity that can lead to death.

The first thing is to be sure in your mind that this risk is worthwhile. Apply the questions set out previously.

The second is if it is worth the risk then let's do all we can to minimize that risk. Patients should be told if a clinician suspects iodine hypersensitivity. The radiologist and radiographer should also be informed of the detailed events that have led to this conclusion. In many circumstances, alternative investigations can be suggested. If an iodine-based contrast examination is essential, there are steps that can be taken to reduce the likelihood of a 'serious untoward event' occurring.

The range of investigations at the radiologist's disposal mean that it is now a rare event to expose a patient with a known hypersensitivity to iodine to an examination requiring an iodine-based contrast medium.

This topic is referred to again in Chapter 2.

Table 1.1 Typical doses from diagnostic medical exposure. (Modified from Royal College of Radiologists handbook, *Making the Best Use of the Radiology Department*, 4th edn.)

Diagnostic procedure	Typical effective dose (mSv)	Equivalent no. of chest X-rays	Approx. equivalent period of natural background radiation
Radiographical examinations			
Limbs and joints (except hip)	<0.01	<0.5	<1.5 days
Chest (single PA film)	0.02	1	3 days
Skull	0.06	3	9 days
Thoracic spine	0.7	35	4 months
Lumbar spine	1	50	5 months
Hip	0.4	20	2 months
Pelvis	0.7	35	4 months
Abdomen	0.7	35	4 months
IVU	2.4	120	14 months
Barium swallow	1.5	75	8 months
Barium meal	2.6	130	15 months
Barium follow-through	3	150	16 months
Barium enema	7.2	360	3.2 years
CT head	2	100	10 months
CT chest	8	400	3.6 years
CT abdomen or pelvis	10	500	4.5 years
Radionuclide studies			
Lung ventilation (^{133}Xe)	0.3	15	7 weeks
Lung perfusion (^{99m}Tc)	1	50	6 months
Bone (^{99m}Tc)	4	200	1.8 years

Abbreviations: CT, computed tomography; IVU, intravenous urogram; PA, posteroanterior.
UK average background radiation = 2.2 mSv/year; regional averages range from 1.5 to 7.5 mSv/year.

Nephrotoxicity (see also Chapter 2)

Contrast media offer a challenge to the kidneys, particularly when injected intra-arterially, and this is dose dependent. The usual half-life of injected contrast is 2 hours. Particular problems arise in the elderly and in dehydrated patients, where the level of renal failure and dehydration are often underestimated. Diabetic patients with mild renal failure are susceptible. These factors mean that patients over 70 years are likely to be at increased risk. Dehydration is also a problem in patients with myeloma.

A number of measures can be taken to prevent contrast media nephrotoxicity if we know about it in advance (e.g. extracellular volume expansion and use of low osmolar contrast media).

It is not uncommon for examination requests to be made when patients are unwell. These are circumstances when the timing of the investigation should be given serious consideration. Of course, on some occasions it is essential to perform an examination immediately, but the additional risk must be recognized and managed.

Alternatively, the reduced benefit of performing an examination quickly with a poor result must be weighed against the benefits of waiting and performing the examination with the patient's condition improved and the imaging circumstances maximized, giving better results. (This applies equally to non-contrast examinations.)

Drug interactions

There are some drugs that interact in an adverse way with contrast media and their excretion. This risk needs to be assessed before booking, not when the patient arrives for an examination. You should at least remember to tell the department before booking if your patient is taking metformin or interferon because of their potential nephrotoxicity (see Chapter 2).

Concurrent administration of nephrotoxic drugs, such as gentamicin, and non-steroidal anti-inflammatory drugs should be avoided.

Asthma

It can be very difficult for the radiologist to tease out whether it is true that a patient has asthma or some other chronic respiratory complaint when he or she arrives at the department for an examination. If the patient is suffering from true asthma and is taking steroids it must be questioned whether a contrast examination is appropriate, as this may provoke an acute exacerbation. If it is, it may be necessary to give further steroid prophylaxis. However, alternative methods of investigation should be considered first.

It is much better for the patient if this issue has been addressed before an appointment is made.

Infection

Sadly, infection is a major cause of concern in modern hospitals, and departments of clinical radiology are no exception.

Patients attending imaging departments expect to be protected from possible cross-infection. In order to do this, those patients with infections, who are a risk to other patients and staff, need to be identified before coming for an appointment or examination (e.g. tuberculosis, hepatitis, methicillin resistant *Staphylococcus aureus* [MRSA]). It beggars belief that wards can nurse MRSA patients in side rooms to protect the rest of the ward patients, but without notification send patients for X-rays that entails them sitting in open waiting areas with other patients — sometimes those from the same ward!

The other side of the coin is that patients who are particularly susceptible to contracting infections (e.g. those with severe lack of immunity) require extra protective measures when particular procedures are carried out.

Staff in the department are also entitled to know when extra risks arise so that additional protective measures can be taken (e.g. HIV infection).

At present, we rely very heavily on the doctors and nurses looking after such patients to inform us, but this does not always happen. It is to be hoped that, in time, such conditions will be highlighted automatically through the electronic record system when a referral is made so the appropriate action can be taken.

Informed consent

Attitudes to informed consent have changed dramatically in the last few years. It is clearly a clinical decision as to how much information is given to a patient but, in general, informed consent means that the patient is in possession of the full facts and that they understand the implications of what is planned for them. When it is necessary to obtain consent in writing is a matter of local policy but it is advisable, when consent has been obtained verbally, that a record of the conversation is made in the patient's notes.

In general, written consent is not required for most radiological examinations but it is required for many interventional procedures. Verbal consent should be obtained for any invasive procedure, which includes intravenous injection.

For interventional procedures such as angioplasty or biopsy, written consent should be obtained by a professional who understands the procedure and its complications fully. Ideally, that person should be capable of performing the procedure. Written information material is very helpful and is widely available.

Do not mislead your patients if you are not sure what a particular procedure entails. You will not be criticized for not knowing, but you will be deemed to be in the wrong if the patient is not fully informed before any act that potentially poses a risk to him or her is undertaken at your behest. Most departments will have well-developed procedures—you just need to learn about them and use them. If in doubt, consult a senior colleague or radiologist.

Pregnancy and the fetus

This issue is covered in Chapter 2.

Confidentiality

You will have received some instruction during your undergraduate years regarding confidentiality and your own behaviour. There is often an expectation that anyone can ring up the radiology department and find out the result of a patient's examination without any safeguards and without any consideration of who else may be within earshot of the phone. Compare this with getting information about your own account at the bank!

Confidentiality applies to all areas.

Using the department

Making referrals

If you regard every request for imaging

as a clinical referral for an expert specialist opinion, you will be taking a large stride towards ensuring that you get the best service from the imaging department for your patients.

Good communication of your patient's details and your expectations is essential. Throughout this book you will be given tips as to where and when this is particularly important. As with many clinical situations, direct conversations can create miracles!

Delegation of responsibility

Radiologists carry the ultimate responsibility for patient care, both legally and clinically, when imaging takes place. In many circumstances this is delegated within protocols to radiographers and technicians. House officers need to understand and recognize these limitations. Do not be surprised if the radiographer wishes to refer to a more senior source. They are not being obstructive but simply keeping to the guidelines that they have to work within. Some referrals have to be made on a consultant to consultant basis in many hospitals. There are good reasons for this.

Guidelines and protocols are developed to provide a framework for all to work within, but they can be varied whenever the individual patient need demands it. Many of these variations can be discussed and agreed at regular clinicoradiological or multidisciplinary meetings and your attendance at these is strongly recommended.

If any situation is proving difficult, referral directly to the radiologist is recommended. A joint discussion between the clinician and radiologist provides the best solution.

Interpretation of the image

Interpretation of the image is usually conducted by a specialist radiologist and a formal report is provided. There will be many circumstances in which a radiologist is not available and you have to rely on your own efforts. When this is the case, remember that it is a requirement under the IRMER legislation to make a record of your interpretation in the notes. Be very careful about the way that you record verbal discussions. If you quote a colleague's opinion in the notes, be sure to check that you have understood them properly. (Note: although radiographers may be very experienced they are not medically qualified — the final responsibility is yours unless you refer to a senior colleague or radiologist.)

Formal interpretation sometimes takes time because of the need to compare with previous examinations, to consult a colleague or to refer to textbooks.

In many cases away from A&E, discussions about patients can take place at regular meetings between clinicians and radiologists. These are highly recommended, both from a patient management point of view but also for everyone's education. The radiologist will learn from the feedback you give them of the final clinical outcome. Do not spare their blushes!

Priorities

It is sometimes difficult for clinicians to understand why their most urgent and important referral is not seen in the same light by the radiology department. It is a constant challenge for staff in imaging departments to arrange lists of patients referred by a number of different clinicians whose sole interest is in their own patients.

If your patient is particularly sick let the radiographer know, so that delays and time spent in the department can be minimized.

The key to success is clear communication of the real need without exaggeration. This applies to out-of-hours requests particularly, when the need for urgent or emergency examination should be clearly understood and agreed by all concerned.

From time to time we all get it wrong.

Audit

Many clinical audit projects require input from imaging departments and vice versa. The data to be used and the mechanisms for collection should be agreed in advance by all parties.

Research

Most hospitals have governance arrangements that need to be followed in order to conduct a piece of research. They should tell you how to arrange for any additional imaging and whether ethical permission is necessary. Managers will need to be involved to sort out any additional funding requirement.

One of the best ways to understand the workings of a radiology department and to see what has to be done to patients to obtain an image (e.g. barium enemas in the elderly and infirm) is to come, visit and see for yourselves. Too many students fail to take up this offer before graduation. If you are one of them, do not hesitate in coming forward now. You will benefit and so will your patients.

Further reading

Burrows EH. *Pioneers and Early Years: A History of British Radiology*. Channel Islands: Colophon, 1986.

Making the Best Use of a Department of Clinical Radiology: Guidelines for Doctors, 5th edn. London: Royal College of Radiologists, 2003.

Chapter 2: **Imaging techniques**

This chapter covers:
• Conventional X-ray (plain film)
• Contrast studies (barium and water-soluble)
• Ultrasound
• Computed tomography
• Magnetic resonance imaging
• Nuclear medicine
• Positron emission tomography
• Picture archiving and communication system

Introduction

There are a number of different imaging modalities that you will become familiar with during medical school and house jobs. Awareness of the relative strengths and weaknesses of these techniques will help you to decide when each should be used. It is important to be aware that some procedures involve ionizing radiation (e.g. conventional X-rays, CT, contrast studies). Always consider before requesting a procedure that involves ionizing radiation:
• Will it effect management?
• Is there an appropriate alternative that does not involve ionizing radiation (e.g. magnetic resonance imaging [MRI] or ultrasound [US])?

These alternatives should particularly be considered in the young, fertile or pregnant. These issues are important in light of the IRMER, which try to limit the utilization of medical radiation. If you are unsure about which examination is appropriate, liaise with the radiology department for advice.

Conventional X-ray (plain film)

This uses a tungsten source to generate X-rays. The X-rays are radiated through the body part of interest and on to a film cassette or digital X-ray camera positioned behind the body part. A special phosphor coating inside the cassette glows and exposes the film. The resulting film is then developed like a photograph. Many departments have a digital X-ray camera rather than film cassette, which contains a similar phosphor and converts the X-rays to an electron beam that drives a TV monitor from which a digital picture can be viewed. This digital image is printed on to film or archived into computer memory.

The resulting image is a two-dimensional representation of a three-dimensional object. It depends on how attenuating to X-rays the tissue of interest is, which is related to the thickness, density and atomic number. It also depends on which tissues are superimposed on each other. The varying attenuations are represented by shades of grey on the film or monitor; white being the most attenuating and black the least. Essentially, there are six different attenuations that you can see on plain films, in order of increasing greyness: air (black); fat and soft tissue; bone; contrast; and metal (white).

You will find that you request certain types of X-ray commonly (e.g. CXR, abdominal X-ray [AXR]), and these will be dealt with later in the book. Some may have a high dose (see Chapter 1 for a range of doses for common procedures involving ionizing radiation). Note the particularly high doses associated with lumbar spine X-ray, CT and barium enema.

Pregnancy and ionizing radiation

Radiation is teratogenic to the fetus so avoid if at all possible in those who are, or may be pregnant (particularly in the first trimester).
• Check with women of reproductive age if they are pregnant or have a delayed period prior to exposure to ionizing radiation. You can use a pregnancy test if you are unsure.
• Delay investigations if possible and let the department know if there is a possibility of pregnancy.
• Use a non-ionizing alternative (MRI, US).
• In emergencies, CT head or CXR gives a relatively low dose to the fetus. Ask for radiological advice if you are unsure.
• Record all decisions in the notes.

Contrast studies

Any two organs of a similar density and average atomic number are indistinguishable on an X-ray. Contrast media are therefore necessary to create an artificial contrast between the organ to be diagnosed and the surrounding tissue. It also opacifies normal tubular structures such as bowel, blood vessels and urinary tract. Contrast is commonly used with fluoroscopic procedures (screening), plain films (intravenous urogram [IVU]) and CT.

All contrast media are based on the principle of a non-toxic suspension or solution that contains a significant proportion of elements with a high atomic number. Barium and water-soluble contrast are the two main agents.

Barium

Barium sulphate is an inert contrast agent used to opacify the gastrointestinal tract. It comes in a variety of suspensions designed for specific purposes. Try to be specific as to which region of the bowel you would like evaluated, as this will dictate the type of barium preparation used. Discuss with the radiologist if you are not sure.

Barium examinations

• Barium swallow.
• Barium meal: rarely performed with the advent of endoscopy (see later in book).
• Small bowel follow-through/enema: used for evaluating small bowel.
• Barium enema.
   Some examinations require a lot of movement (barium meals and enemas) and may not be appropriate in the frail or elderly. Consider alternative investigations such as colonoscopy or CT.

Important points

• Barium is contraindicated in suspected perforation (causes a high-mortality peritonitis or mediastinitis). Suspected perforation is an indication for a water-soluble agent.

• Aspiration may occur during barium swallow and requires urgent physiotherapy. Arrange the same day.

• Barium enema is contraindicated if a deep rectal biopsy has been performed via rigid scope within the previous 5 days.

• Large bowel barium studies require preparation. Laxatives used for barium enemas can cause dehydration. Consider admission for preparation in the elderly and infirm.

• Barium causes artefact on CT, making it difficult to interpret. This will delay use of CT by up to 2 weeks.

Water-soluble contrast agents

These are iodine-based clear viscous liquids. They can be classified into the older ionic and newer non-ionic agents. Ionic agents, although cheap, have a far higher incidence of side-effects and are no longer used intravenously.

Uses of ionic contrast agents (e.g. Gastrografin, Urografin)

• For large bowel evaluation rectally in patients with suspected perforation or at risk of perforation (e.g. colitis).

• Can be injected into T-tube, into a fistula (fistulogram) or sinus (sinogram).

• To check for leaks from an ileal pouch or bowel anastomosis.

• Only used orally as a dilute bowel preparation in CT. They cause a chemical pneumonitis if aspirated.

Uses of non-ionic contrast agents

• Can be injected intravenously (e.g. IVU, CT) or intra-arterially (e.g. angiogram).

• Contrast swallows in suspected perforation or in children.

Side-effects of water-soluble contrast agents

• *Nephrotoxicity following intravenous injection* (avoid these studies in renal impairment):
 – Increased risk in renal impairment, diabetes mellitus, dehydration, in the elderly and myeloma.
 – Where appropriate include details of the patient's renal function on the request form if requesting a procedure that may need intravenous contrast.

• *Metformin and intravenous contrast:*
 – These patients are at risk of lactic acidosis after intravenous contrast administration.
 – Check renal function before procedure. If it is abnormal patients should not be on metformin anyway (remember it is renally excreted).
 – Metformin should be stopped before and for a period after intravenous contrast (check individual department for protocol). Do not restart unless renal function is normal.

• *Anaphylactic reactions:*
 – Let the department know if there is a history of iodine allergy.
 – Reactions include rash and wheeze. Severe reactions are rare (1 in 1000), as is death (1 in 12 000–40 000).
 – Premedication with steroids is sometimes used in those with previous reactions or at high risk, but liaise with the department.

• *Extravasation/phlebitis at injection site.*

Ultrasound

This uses ultra-high-frequency sound waves generated from a transducer in the US probe, which penetrates tissues and is reflected back. An image is created, depending on the reflecting and absorbing properties of tissue. The image is displayed as a grey scale on a monitor. Objects appear as bright (hyperechoic, e.g. gallstones) if highly reflective or as dark (hypoechoic, e.g. water) if sound passes freely through. Isoechoic structures are similar in appearance to surrounding tissue. Doppler US is a useful adjunct, which estimates velocity of moving structures and has vascular applications. Patient preparation is often required, especially in the upper abdomen — liaise with the department.

Advantages of US

• No ionizing radiation.
• Portable and can image in any plane.
• Real time: good for mobile structures (e.g. heart valves) and guiding drainage or biopsy procedures.
• US has a wide range of applications but is particularly useful in obstetrics, children and vascular evaluation.

Disadvantages of US

• Operator dependent.
• Limited by body habitus, poor visualization of deep structures in the obese.
• US cannot scan through gas. This is a particular problem in the abdomen with excess bowel gas. The pancreas and retroperitoneum in particular are often obscured.
• US cannot penetrate through bone.

Computed tomography

Modern scanners consists of a rotating beam of high-energy X-rays and a 360° array of detectors. The patient slides through this rotating array and the resulting image is a series of vertical slices, representing the varying densities of tissue across the slice in the patient. A detailed knowledge of cross-sectional anatomy is required for interpretation of these images.

The density of an object on a CT scan is measured relative to water in Hounsfield units ranging from approximately −1000 (air: low density) to +1000 (bone: high density). As there are about 2000 different Hounsfield numbers and the human eye can only appreciate about 10–15 different grey scales, scans are windowed according to the particular type of tissue that needs to be examined. This improves the contrast between tissues and this is the advantage of CT over other imaging modalities. The common windows most used are lung, soft tissue, brain and bone.

The image is displayed on a grey scale with more dense matter appearing as white (bone, blood), less dense matter as black (air, fat), and soft tissue appearing as shades of grey. Most CT images in this book are on soft-tissue windows but examples of lung window (Chapter 3, Fig. 3.4a) and bone window (Chapter 12 Fig. 12.2) images are included.

Images can be obtained rapidly (e.g. a single breath hold for the whole chest).

Modern scanners have a high enough resolution to perform angiography after an intravenous injection of contrast. They can also scan an entire volume of a patient (e.g. knee) and this can be viewed in any plane, which is useful in orthopaedics, as a three-dimensional image.

Patient preparation

Different departments have varying protocols. Abdominal and pelvic examinations usually need oral contrast (dilute ionic) for bowel opacification and intravenous non-ionic contrast for opacification of vasculature and viscera. Remember previous comments about iodine allergy and renal impairment. The patient may need to tolerate oral contrast. Lack of oral contrast may limit the accuracy of the examination. Consider this if your patient is vomiting or nil by mouth (NBM) (for example suspected perforation, or for an acute abdominal problem that may need surgery).

Advantages of CT

• Good contrast between tissues and useful in assessment of abdomen, retroperitoneum, pelvis and mediastinum.
• Not degraded by bowel gas.
• Highly sensitive in detecting intracranial blood.

Disadvantages of CT

• CT is a relatively high-dose procedure (see Chapter 1).
• Recent barium studies obscure images of the abdomen and pelvis. There may have to be a 2-week delay between studies. Bear this in mind if CT may be required for your patient.
• Artefact is caused by high-density metal in teeth and joint replacements. This may limit the diagnostic accuracy of neck and pelvic examinations.
• It may be difficult to scan dense bony areas for the same reason (e.g. posterior fossa).

• The accuracy of CT is limited if the patient cannot hold his or her breath or lie still.
• Most CT scanners have size and weight limits.

Magnetic resonance imaging

All hydrogen nuclei have a physical property called a magnetic moment or spin if they are put in a strong magnetic field. When combined with an electromagnetic pulse this produces a signal, which can be measured, and an image generated. Each slice of the MR image is essentially a map of the distribution of this property of hydrogen nuclei in the various tissues of the body.

The main sequences are T1 and T2. T1-weighted sequences show fluid as low signal (dark) and fat as high signal (white). On T2 weighting, fat is high signal and fluid is very high signal. A STIR sequence can be used to suppress fat and highlight oedema changes in tissues.

Gadolinium-based contrast is a non-iodine-based paramagnetic compound, sometimes used to alter the T1 signal of tissues to aid diagnosis. Although apparently not nephrotoxic, it should be used with caution in renal impairment.

Advantages of MRI

• No ionizing radiation.
• Multiplanar capabilities.
• High-resolution high-contrast images of the internal organs.
• Widely used in brain, spine and joint imaging.
• Useful in bony areas such as the spine and posterior fossa and pelvis, where CT is often limited.

• Magnetic resonance angiography (MRA) or venography can be performed without contrast injection (useful in those who have an iodine allergy or renal impairment).

Disadvantages of MRI

• Systems are expensive and not widely available.
• Scanners are noisy and the patient may have to stay still for a long period of time. If they move, part of the scan may have to be repeated.
• High incidence (up to 10%) of scan failure resulting from claustrophobia. The incidence of this is decreasing in newer, more open machines.
• Orthopaedic hardware (screws, plates, artificial joints) in the area of a scan can cause severe artefact.
• Not as sensitive in detecting blood in acute cerebral trauma.

Contraindications

These are related to the strong central magnetic field and the ability to move ferromagnetic objects at considerable speed. Patients with the following should not enter the scanning room:
• Pacemaker
• Aneurysm clip
• Metallic heart valve
• Cochlear, otological or ear implant
• In those who work with metal or who have had a shrapnel injury.

Some surgical prostheses (e.g. screws, rods and plates) need a waiting period of at least 6 weeks after surgery to allow for postoperative fibrosis before scanning.

Always consult with the MR department about device safety. Newer prostheses may not be ferromagnetic and hence safe in the scanner.

Nuclear medicine

Nuclear medicine (NM) provides functional information but relatively poor anatomical detail. It uses physiologically active molecules, which are labelled with radionuclide (a molecule that emits radioactivity). For example methylene diphosphonate (MDP) labelled with technetium (^{99m}Tc). The labelled molecule is called a radiopharmaceutical. Technetium is the most commonly used radionuclide and emits gamma rays.

The radiopharmaceuticals are injected (e.g. bone scan) or inhaled (ventilation/perfusion scan) and allowed to distribute where these molecules are normally utilized (e.g. the osteoblasts in bone in the case of ^{99m}Tc MDP in bone scans). The distribution and concentration of these molecules in the body can be detected by the radiation emitted by the radionuclide, which is detected by a device called the gamma camera. A grey scale image is generated, showing the concentration and distribution of the radiopharmaceutical in the body.

Advantages of NM

• Provides functional information.
• Can be used safely in renal impairment.

Disadvantages of NM

• Poor anatomical resolution.
• High dose (see Table 1.1).
• Some examinations may be limited by availability of radionuclides.
• Patients may need to lie relatively still for long periods.

Positron emission tomography

There are only a handful of institutions that can perform positron emission tomography (PET). It uses positron (a positive electron) emitting radionuclides, labelled on to metabolically active molecules; 18 fluorine-fluorodeoxyglucose being most commonly used. This is injected and is taken up in proportion to the metabolic activity of the tissue. Very metabolically active tissues, such as cancers, take it up avidly. The positrons generate two high-energy gamma rays at 180° to each other. This allows accurate localization by detectors on a dual-headed PET scanner to visualize the distribution of this metabolically active tissue. It is used commonly in staging of lung cancer, melanoma and lymphoma.

Picture archiving and communication system

These are computer-based systems, which eliminate film. If your hospital has a picture archiving and communication system (PACS), all of the imaging modalities mentioned may be stored on computer memory, which can be viewed as and when required on a computer monitor rather than printed on to conventional plain film. These systems consist of:

• *Computer memory:* storage device (a large amount of long- and short-term memory).

• *Computerized radiography:* taking images in a digital format so that they can be stored on a computer memory. This is relatively easy for CT, MR and US, where the images are generated by computers. Many institutions are now also taking plain films with digital X-ray cameras.

• *Monitors and viewing software:* for viewing and manipulating image contrast, size and serial comparison.

• *Network:* to send the images to where you want to see them in the hospital.

Advantages of PACS

• Easier access.
• Cost saving.
• No more lost films.

Disadvantages of PACS

• Initial cost.
• System failure visible and catastrophic.
• Reduced discussion between radiologists and clinicians.

Further reading

Making the Best Use of a Department of Clinical Radiology: Guidelines for Doctors, 5th edn. London: Royal College of Radiologists, 2003.

Thomsen HS, Morcos SK. Contrast media and the kidney: European Society of Urogenital Radiology [ESUR] guidelines. *British Journal of Radiology* 2003; **76**: 513–18.

Chapter 3: **Respiratory system**

This chapter covers:
Common conditions
• Lung cancer, lung metastases, lymphangitis carcinomatosa
• Chronic obstructive pulmonary disease, sarcoidosis, tuberculosis, bronchiectasis
• Common clinical findings: pleural effusion, pneumothorax, pneumonia
• Asbestos-related lung disease, interstitial fibrosis
Common presentations in which imaging can help
Symptoms of lung disease are not often disease-specific and include:
• Shortness of breath
• Chest pain, either pleuritic or non-pleuritic
• Haemoptysis is a symptom that requires investigation: common causes include lung cancer and tuberculosis
• Productive cough is common with acute infection and chronically is a characteristic feature of bronchiectasis
• Dry cough is present in many conditions, including interstitial fibrosis
• Wheeze is a non-specific symptom characteristic of asthma but also seen in other conditions such as heart failure, inhaled foreign bodies and some central lung cancers

Imaging strategy

CXR

Indications

One of the most common requests you will make will be for a CXR. A list of indications would be very long and not very useful, so the best approach to determining whether to request a CXR is to ask yourself how it will change your management of the patient. If it will alter management, then it is justified.

Standard views

PA

A standard CXR is performed with the patient standing facing the X-ray cassette, which contains film or computerized radiography plate. The X-ray source is behind the patient at a fixed distance. The X-ray beam passes from posterior to anterior (PA). This technique minimizes magnification of anterior structures. The size of the heart and mediastinal structures can be assessed on a PA image and compared to similar previous examinations.

AP

If the patient is too ill or immobile to obtain an erect PA view, an AP film can be obtained. The X-ray cassette is placed behind the patient. The X-ray beam passes from anterior to posterior (AP).

The patient will often be lying on a trolley or a bed and this causes magnification of anterior structures by a variable degree so an accurate assessment of the size of the heart and aorta cannot be made, although if they look normal in size, they are!

Lateral

Lateral chest films are of limited value, and tend to be over-requested. They are useful for the assessment of areas hidden on a PA film by the diaphragm, heart or bone. Ask a radiologist for advice.

US

This is a valuable technique in the assessment of the size and position of pleural effusions, and can be used to guide aspiration of pleural fluid. It can be particularly useful if loculation of the fluid has occurred because of previous disease or intervention.

CT

Two types of scan of the chest are performed for assessment of lung disease: standard and high-resolution CT (HRCT) scans.

Standard scans with intravenous (IV) contrast are used to stage lung tumours, investigate lung masses and to assess the mediastinum and pleura. They are also performed in the staging of other malignancies to detect metastases or assess sites of involvement in lymphomas.

High-resolution scans demonstrate fine detail of the lung structure and are used in the assessment of interstitial lung disease and air-space disease. Air-space disease involves the lumen of the bronchial tree and is usually in the alveoli, as is seen, for example, in pneumonia and pulmonary oedema. Interstitial diseases involve the lung structure (e.g. sarcoidosis, some pneumonias and interstitial fibrosis). Characteristic patterns of involvement are often seen on HRCT and a firm diagnosis can often be made.

The radiologist/radiographer will need to decide which technique to use in advance and therefore needs to be fully informed of the clinical problem to be addressed.

PET

This is a highly specialized investigation performed in a few centres only. The technique identifies areas of increased glucose metabolism and, as malignant lung tumours have high levels of glucose metabolism, PET scanning is used for staging prior to surgery and for follow-up when available.

MRI

This has only a limited role at the present time. It is sometimes useful in assessing brachial plexus and chest wall involvement by tumours, although the patient's symptoms are often the most reliable evidence of chest wall involvement.

Carcinoma of the lung

Clinical presentation

Common clinical presentations of primary tumour are:
• A coincidental finding of a mass on CXR

• Cough, haemoptysis, wheeze, pneumonia: often indicative of a central tumour
• Pleuritic chest pain, brachial plexus pain and/or Horner's syndrome (Pancoast's tumour) that may suggest a peripheral tumour
• More general symptoms (e.g. shortness of breath, cough)
• Paraneoplastic syndromes (e.g. inappropriate antidiuretic hormone secretion), non-metastatic neuromyopathic pain, clubbing and hypertrophic osteoarthropathy, thrombophlebitis migrans and cachexia
• Metastatic disease, depending on the site (e.g. brain or bone).

If you suspect that your patient may have carcinoma of the lung, initial investigations will be determined by the appearances of the CXR.

Appearance on CXR

Common appearances seen on CXR are:
• *Lung mass:* varying in size and shape, with or without cavitation. Peripheral consolidation or collapse may occur distal to a central stenosing tumour. A slowly enlarging cavitating mass is a classic presentation of a squamous cell carcinoma of the lung (Fig. 3.1).
• *Non-surgical lobar collapse in adults:* look for localized central bulging of the

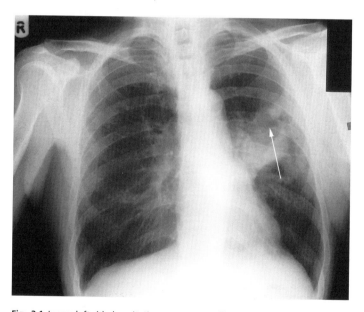

Fig. 3.1 Large left-sided cavitating squamous cell carcinoma is present, which contains an air–fluid level (white arrow).

collapsed lobe, as this may be a tumour (S–sign of Golden; see Fig. 3.2).

• *Pleural effusion:* a large unilateral pleural effusion may mask an underlying tumour.

Tips

• Always look for any associated features that will confirm the diagnosis of malignancy, such as evidence of local

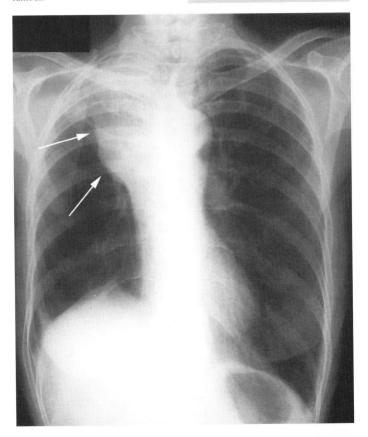

Fig. 3.2 Right upper lobe collapse secondary to a central occluding carcinoma. Note the trachea is deviated to the right with the right hilum elevated and not visualized, consistent with right upper lobe volume loss. There is characteristic convex bulging of the border of the collapsed right upper lobe due to an obstructing tumour (white arrows), the so-called S-sign of Golden.

chest wall or bone invasion (Fig. 3.3), metastases in the lungs or bones, enlarged hilar and/or mediastinal nodes.

- Always suspect a central bronchogenic tumour if a patient presents with lobar collapse, if pneumonia does not clear or if pneumonia arises in the upper lobes.
- Always check the apical regions of the lungs carefully.
- An unusual presentation is that of patchy or confluent nodules and/or consolidation unilaterally or bilaterally seen in broncho-alveolar cell carcinoma (<6% of lung carcinomas but may be increasing in incidence).

Further investigations

- *Bronchoscopy:* useful to obtain a tissue diagnosis, particularly for central lesions.
- *CT scan for preoperative staging* (Fig. 3.4a,b): staging will assess the size of the primary tumour, hilar and mediastinal node involvement and the presence of distant metastases in the liver or adrenals. Assessment of involvement of central structures (important if surgery is contemplated) such as the pulmonary arteries, main bronchi and heart will also be made.
- *CT and CT-guided biopsy*: for cases where knowing the tissue type will affect management. This usually arises when

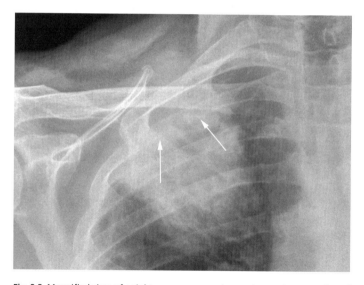

Fig. 3.3 Magnified view of a right upper zone carcinoma demonstrates erosion of the inferior cortical margin of the posterior third rib (arrows).

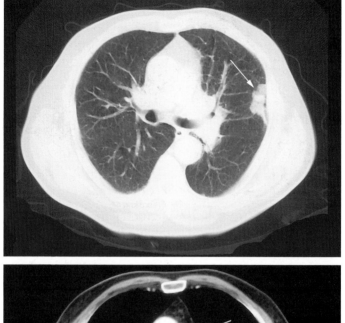

a

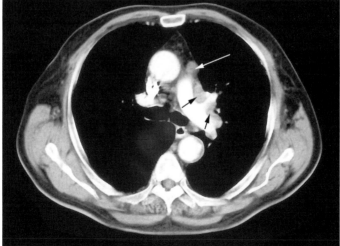

b

Fig. 3.4 (a) An axial CT section on lung window settings demonstrates a peripheral carcinoma in the left upper lobe (white arrow). (b) In the same patient as (a), post-contrast CT on mediastinal windows demonstrates enlarged nodes at the aorto-pulmonary window (white arrow) and the left hilum (black arrows).

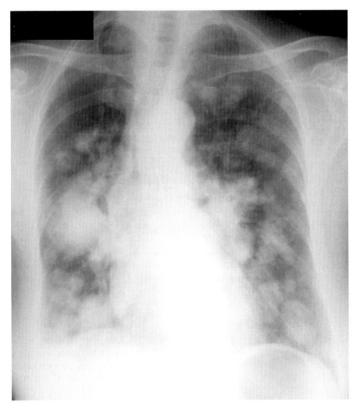

Fig. 3.5 Widespread soft-tissue metastases (cannon ball) of varying size are demonstrated throughout both lungs in a patient with metastatic carcinoma of the colon.

Table 3.1 Useful information regarding patients referred for lung or pleural biopsy.

Can be used for:
Focal lung lesions >8 mm diameter, depending on site of lesion
Focal pleural lesions or diffuse pleural thickening

Contraindications
Patient unable to give informed consent or unable to cooperate
Bleeding diathesis
Severe COPD/emphysema unable to withstand pneumothorax — ask the chest physician!

Patient preparation
Nil by mouth (4 hr)
Intravenous access
Consent
Coagulation screen

Complications
Haemoptysis as a result of intrapulmonary haemorrhage
Pneumothorax. Small pneumothoraces are common. Aspiration and/or chest drain are rarely needed

the primary tumour has been shown to be inoperable on CT scanning (Table 3.1).
• *PET:* to aid diagnosis and to stage distant nodes prior to surgery.

Lung metastases

The lungs are a common site of haematogenous metastatic disease. Common primary sites include:
• Breast
• Kidney
• Head and neck
• Colorectal.

CXR

Several patterns are seen:
• *Nodules:* one or more of varying sizes (Fig. 3.5)
• *Poorly defined soft-tissue masses*
• *Miliary metastases:* tiny widespread soft-tissue metastatic nodules, all of similar size.

Comparison with previous films or reference to previous reports is often rewarding.

CT

CT may be useful if there is doubt on the CXR. It is a very sensitive technique and often demonstrates more metastases than are visible on the CXR, even in retrospect!

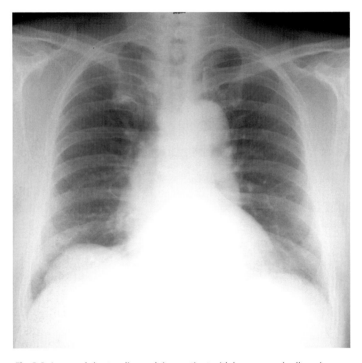

Fig. 3.6 A normal chest radiograph in a patient with known renal cell carcinoma.

Lymphangitis carcinomatosa

Involvement of the central lymphatic channels of the chest by metastatic disease results in lymphangitis carcinomatosa, whether the primary tumour is in the chest or remote. Common primary sites producing lymphangitis carcinomatosa are breast, cervix, lung, pancreas, prostate, stomach and thyroid.

Changes become apparent in advanced cases on CXR and on CT scanning.

CXR

CXR may show (Figs 3.6 & 3.7):
- Reticulation and irregular septal lines
- Soft–tissue nodular densities
- Enlarged hilar nodes (< 50%)
- Enlarged mediastinal nodes
- Unilateral or bilateral distribution
- Pleural effusions.

CT

HRCT is valuable in establishing the diagnosis of lymphangitis carcinomatosa

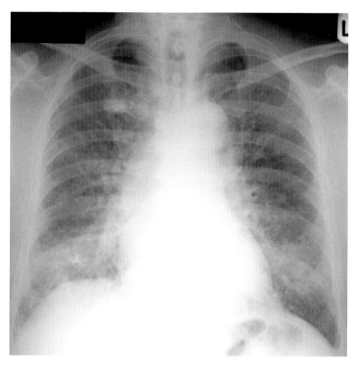

Fig. 3.7 Two months later, the same patient as in Fig. 3.6 developed symptoms of shortness of breath with evidence of lymphangitis carcinomatosa on CXR. There are diffuse infiltrates within the lungs.

if there is uncertainty over the CXR appearances.

Chronic obstructive pulmonary disease

The term chronic obstructive pulmonary disease (COPD) is used to describe what is often a combination of chronic bronchitis and emphysema.

These clinical syndromes lead to chronic, mostly irreversible, airways obstruction. Symptoms include chronic cough, sputum production and shortness of breath.

Emphysema

Emphysema is a condition in which there are permanently enlarged air spaces distal to the terminal bronchioles, with destruction of the alveolar walls, often as a result of smoking but also seen as a result of α_1-antitrypsin deficiency. This leads to inefficient gas exchange.

Imaging is indicated at first presentation. It is only indicated for follow-up if there is a significant change in symptoms or signs.

CXR

Moderate to severe emphysema can be diagnosed but mild emphysema is often overlooked, even by radiologists.
• *Large volume lungs* (Fig. 3.8):
 – Low flat diaphragm
 – Visibility of the anterior end of the seventh rib above the diaphragm
 – If a lateral CXR has been performed for another reason, widening of the space (> 2.5 cm) between the ascending aorta and the sternum may be seen
 – Barrel-shaped chest.
• *Bullae:* thin-walled (< 1 mm) air spaces as a result of destruction of alveolar walls (not always associated with significant emphysema elsewhere in the lungs).
• *Reduced vascularity:* found in areas most severely affected and may only be recognized by a radiologist.

Pitfall

It may be difficult to distinguish apical bullae and pneumothorax. Look at the shape of the superior border of the lung. If it is convex superiorly and remains convex at the lateral margin, this is characteristic of a pneumothorax. An apical bulla, where the superior wall of the bulla may be difficult to see, will characteristically result in a concave shape of the superior margin of the lung. If in doubt seek advice.

CT

Only indicated if reduction surgery of bullae is being considered.

Chronic bronchitis

This is a clinical diagnosis based on the symptoms of chronic cough with sputum production, dyspnoea and typical lung function tests. There are no reliable radiographical features of this condition but it is associated with large volume lungs, scarring and intermittent consolidation in acute exacerbations.

Asthma

CXR is not indicated routinely for asthma. However, it is of value if you suspect that there may be a pneumothorax present. Asthma is one of the most common causes of spontaneous pneumothorax as a result of lung disease.

Bronchiectasis

This is defined as localized irreversible dilatation of the bronchial tree. There are many causes of bronchiectasis, the more common ones are:
• Infection (e.g. *Staphylococcus*, tuberculosis, *Klebsiella*, fungal infections)
• Congenital causes (e.g. α_1-antitrypsin deficiency, cystic fibrosis, Kartagener's syndrome, Marfan's syndrome)
• Allergic bronchopulmonary aspergillosis
• Immunodeficiency states.
However, in 40% of cases a cause is not identified.
 Symptoms include:

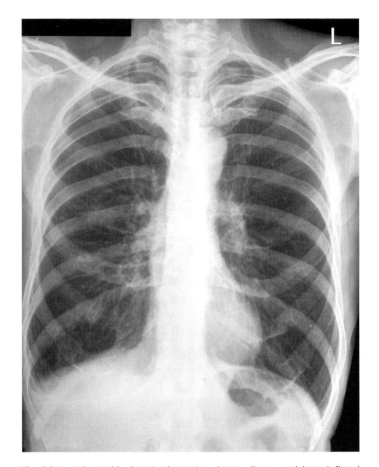

Fig. 3.8 A patient with chronic obstructive airways disease and hyperinflated lungs. The lungs appear hyperlucent, with the diaphragm flattened and eight ribs can be visualized anteriorly in the lung fields.

- Chronic, productive cough
- Recurrent infection
- Dyspnoea
- Haemoptysis.

CXR

The changes may be subtle.
- May appear normal.

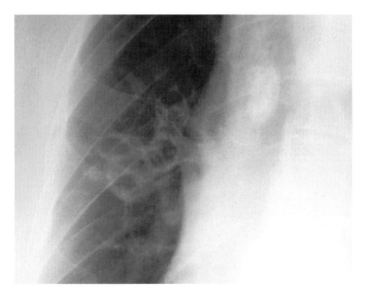

Fig. 3.9 A magnification view of the right mid zone demonstrates thick-walled ring shadows typical of bronchiectasis. These ring densities are caused by thickened bronchi seen end on.

• Bronchial dilatation may be seen as large rings or cyst-like spaces, which may or may not contain fluid levels.
• Bronchial wall thickening may be seen as rings (wall thickness of a few millimetres) or tramlines (parallel walls of bronchi with no tapering). Note the group of rings seen in the right mid zone on the CXR in Fig. 3.9.

CT

CT is indicated in cases with a good clinical history of bronchiectasis with an apparently normal CXR. In cases with abnormal CXR, CT is used if surgery is being contemplated, to demonstrate the extent of involvement.

Sarcoidosis

This is a common disease of unknown origin but immunologically mediated, typified by non-caseating granulomatous lesions affecting many organs. Thoracic disease is present in 90% of cases. The most common involvement is lymph node involvement (43%). Lymph node involvement and lung parenchy-

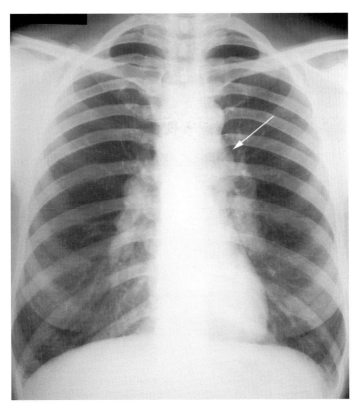

Fig. 3.10 Mediastinal nodal (white arrow) and bilateral hilar nodal enlargement in a patient with sarcoidosis.

mal is seen in approximately 41%. Parenchymal disease alone occurs in approximately 16% of cases.

Presenting clinical features are:
• Asymptomatic
• Erythema nodosum, fever, malaise, joint pains
• Unproductive cough and dyspnoea tend to occur with the more chronic

phase of lung involvement. Wheeze may occur in acute cases.

CXR

The most common finding in the acute phase is the presence of bilateral hilar lymph node enlargement (Fig. 3.10). Check the hilar regions carefully, as small changes can easily be missed. Right paratracheal nodal enlargement is not uncommon. Also:

• Parenchymal disease may occur (43%), characteristically producing reticulonodular changes in the mid and lower zones, which may progress to fibrosis in the mid to upper zones.

• Confluent changes similar to consolidation in the lungs.

• Complete resolution of the early parenchymal changes occurs in one-third of cases; improvement occurs in another 30%.

• Fibrosis is irreversible.

Note:
Pleural effusions are rare (2%)
Cavitation is rare (0.6%)

CT

This may be useful in confirming parenchymal changes and mediastinal lymph node involvement. The parenchymal changes on HRCT are reasonably specific.

Tuberculosis

Active infection with *Mycobacterium tuberculosis* is not common in fit people from countries with an immunization programme, but do be aware of this possibility in patients from abroad or those with reduced immunity. Atypical infection is increasing in incidence.

If a patient has a productive cough and there is a high clinical suspicion of tuberculosis (TB), this information should be conveyed to the radiological staff to allow appropriate management in the department. This applies also to patients referred for follow-up films while in the active stage.

Common symptoms include:
• Cough, haemoptysis
• Shortness of breath
• Weight loss
• Night sweats.

CXR

Reactivated TB (post-primary TB) is the most common form. Features include:
• Consolidation (80%), usually upper lobe or apical segment of lower lobe
• Cavity formation (Fig. 3.11)
• Soft-tissue stranding towards the hilum
• Nodular pattern (20%)
• May see pre-existing calcification in cases of reactivation
• Pleural effusion.

Primary TB is uncommon, but occurs in patients from abroad and those with reduced immunity. CXR features include:
• Consolidation (may be multiple sites)
• Nodules of soft-tissue density
• Hilar and/or mediastinal node enlargement
• Pleural effusion.

Miliary TB may be primary or post-primary, and is characterized by fine soft-tissue nodules throughout lungs of uniform size (2–3 mm) on the CXR.

Note:
Miliary TB does not calcify

Pleural effusions

Effusions may be:
• Transudates, the most common causes are:
  – Congestive cardiac failure
  – Hypoalbuminaemic states (e.g. nephrotic syndrome, cirrhosis).

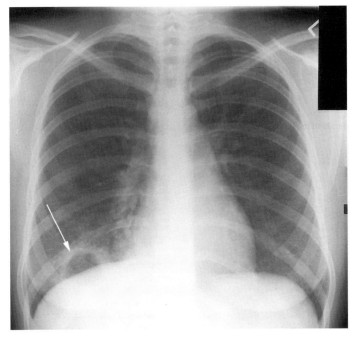

Fig. 3.11 There is a thick-walled cavity (white arrow) seen within an area of tuberculous consolidation in the right lower zone.

- Exudates, the most common causes are:
  - Malignancy
  - Infection
  - Pulmonary emboli (often bloody)
  - Trauma (often bloody, may be chylous).

CXR

PA erect film changes are:
- Blunting of the costophrenic angle
- Meniscus effect in the pleural space
- With large unilateral effusions, shift of the mediastinum to the opposite side of the chest
- Collapse of the underlying lobe or lung
- If loculation occurs as a result of pleural tethering and thickening, lobular 'masses' may be seen, which can be difficult to differentiate from pleural deposits or intrapulmonary masses. A lateral image may be helpful in differentiating the two conditions.

Fluid may track into fissures where loculation may occur, giving rise to apparent intrapulmonary masses (Fig. 3.12).

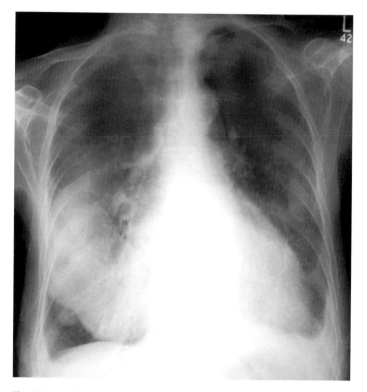

Fig. 3.12 On a frontal chest radiograph, in a patient with cardiac failure, there is evidence of cardiomegaly with small bilateral basal pleural effusions and a large apparent mass identified in the right lower zone. The upper margin of this is not well defined. This represents encysted pleural fluid in the oblique fissure and this can be confirmed on a lateral view.

Subpulmonary effusion is a collection of pleural fluid appearing to be trapped between the lung and the diaphragm. The result is that on a PA film the diaphragm appears flattened and elevated but the apparent dome of the diaphragm lies more laterally than normal. If the effusion is on the left, there will be widening of the space between the 'diaphragm' (top of the effusion) and the stomach bubble.

Always check the costophrenic angles on CXR as this is an area where pathology is easily overlooked.

US

US is useful for confirming the presence of an effusion, assessing its size and marking the site of the effusion prior to aspiration. It is particularly useful where the CXR fails in the recumbent patient.

CT

CT is usually only performed as part of trauma work-up or in cases of empyema to assess how thick the pleura has become prior to possible surgical intervention. It is valuable in looking at the underlying lung and mediastinum in cases of suspected malignancy.

Both CT and US are used to direct the insertion of needles and catheters into loculated effusions.

Pneumothorax

Patients with a pneumothorax commonly present with pleuritic chest pain, with or without shortness of breath.

Common causes

- Spontaneous:
  - *Idiopathic* (80%): caused by the rupture of subpleural blebs in the apices, typically in tall thin young men
  - *Secondary to underlying lung disease*

(20%): the most common underlying lung condition is COPD.
- Traumatic:
  - This may occur as a result of blunt or penetrating trauma
  - Iatrogenic causes include positive pressure ventilation, insertion of a central venous line or pacemaker.

CXR

Standard inspiratory PA image

Look for a peripheral area where no lung markings are visible and try to identify the lung border to assess the size of the pneumothorax.

In addition to the air in the pleural space, you may see varying degrees of collapse of the underlying lung, from small subsegmental areas (often linear or triangular) to collapse of the whole of one or more lobes.

Expiratory image

If you have a high clinical suspicion of a pneumothorax and cannot see one on the standard inspiratory film, then an expiratory film may be helpful as the pneumothorax will be larger and the lung will appear more opaque than on the inspiratory film, thus accentuating the difference in density between the lung and the pneumothorax.

Pitfalls

- Differentiation from emphysematous bullae.
- Skin folds may mimic the edge of a lung but you will still be able to see lung markings peripheral to the fold.

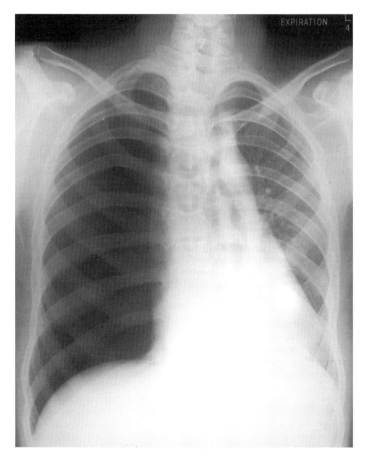

Fig. 3.13 There is a large right-sided pneumothorax, which is under tension with mediastinal shift to the left. This occurred spontaneously.

Tension pneumothorax

This is a medical emergency requiring rapid intervention, usually dramatically improved by the insertion of a chest drain. If there is no clinical doubt about the diagnosis and the patient is critically ill, it may be necessary to insert a chest drain or needle prior to any imaging.

In cases of tension pneumothorax, air

passes into the pleural space on inspiration, but on expiration air is trapped in the pleural space, usually as a result of a ball valve effect. The result is the steady increase in the size of the pneumothorax. With each breath the diaphragm on the affected side is flattened and the lung on the affected side collapses. Rising pressure causes shift of the mediastinum to the opposite side (Fig. 3.13). This eventually leads to 'kinking' of the trachea and sudden obstruction that may be fatal. Urgent action is required.

Acute pneumonia

Acute infection of the lung, as opposed to the bronchi, produces pneumonia in which exudate replaces air in the alveoli leading to radiological sign of consolidation. However, most mild cases of pneumonia are acquired in the community and treated successfully by general practitioners without resorting to chest radiography. A CXR taken acutely in A&E when the diagnosis is obvious is unnecessary and may be misleading if performed before the exudate has formed. A CXR is very valuable in cases where there is clinical doubt or failure to recover satisfactorily.

The changes of pneumonia on CXR are:
- Peripheral soft-tissue density shadowing: consolidation (Fig. 3.14)
- Air in branching bronchi and bronchioles within this shadowing: the air bronchogram (Fig. 3.14)
- Pleural effusion.

Note:
Pneumonia may be the result of a lesion causing narrowing of a proximal bronchus. Depending on age and circumstances, the most common causes are carcinoma and foreign body.

Any transudate or exudate (e.g. blood, pulmonary oedema) in the alveoli will have exactly the same appearance on CXR (consolidation).

Patterns of involvement may help to point to certain organisms as the cause:
- Lobar pneumonia involves the whole or major part of a lobe:
  - The lobe involved can usually be determined on a PA chest film alone using the silhouette sign
  - Typical organisms are *Streptococcus pneumoniae*, *Klebsiella* and *Mycoplasma*.
- Bronchopneumonia involves the large airways as well as parts of the lung:
  - Consolidation is patchy and an air bronchogram may not be present
  - There is also an interstitial element to the changes that may be evident on a CXR. This pattern may show nodularity or ring shadows
  - Typical organisms are *Staphylococcus*, *Streptococcus*, Gram-negative infections
  - In immunocompromised patients, consider also fungi, *Legionella* and *Aspergillus*.
- Extensive bilateral pneumonia is unusual and should alert you to:
  - Viral infections or *Legionella*
  - In immunocompromised patients, consider pneumocystis, fungi and tuberculosis.

Lung abscess

This is one of the possible complications of infection and may arise *de novo* or as a

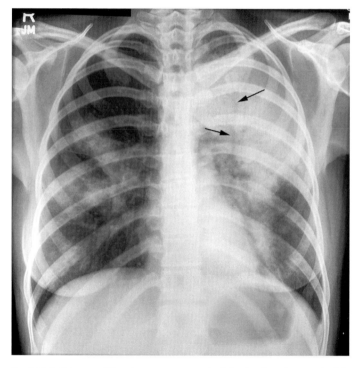

Fig. 3.14 In this case of *Streptococcus pneumoniae* infection there is extensive left upper lobe consolidation with some patchy consolidation also in the right mid zone. Note the prominent air bronchogram seen in the consolidated left upper lobe (black arrows), which is a result of normal bronchus being outlined by consolidated lung.

complication of pneumonic consolidations. If arising from an area of pneumonia, look for an air-filled cavity or fluid level in the area of consolidation. If arising *de novo*, it may appear as a 'mass lesion'. Again, look carefully for air or fluid level within the mass.

These changes may represent a gas-forming organism or suggest a bronchial connection. A direct specimen for microbiology (under CT guidance) is often helpful if blood cultures are negative.

Remember that cavitation is also seen in other conditions (e.g. malignancy, both primary and secondary, pulmonary emboli and rheumatoid nodules).

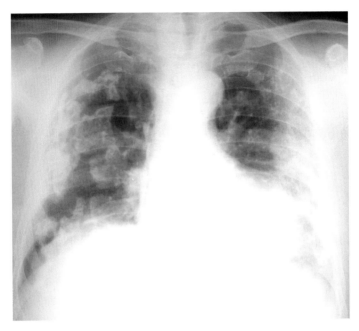

Fig. 3.15 This patient has widespread pleural calcifications secondary to previous asbestos exposure.

Asbestos-related lung disease

Inhalation of asbestos fibres, particularly amosite (brown asbestos) and crocidolite (blue–black asbestos) is an industrial hazard that can lead to chest disease. Patients may be entitled to compensation.

Disease categories

Benign pleural disease

Pleural effusions may develop after a latent period averaging 10 years after exposure. Pleural plaques and pleural calcification occur typically on the diaphragm or posterolaterally on the PA films. They are often asymptomatic (Fig. 3.15).

Malignant mesothelioma

This can develop in the pleura, usually unilaterally. Five to 10% of asbestos workers develop malignant mesothelioma. It has a latent period of 20–45 years. The most common presenting symptom is chest pain, which is usually non-pleuritic. Diffuse progressive thickening of the pleura on one side is shown on CXR or CT. Evidence of chest wall invasion (rib destruction or soft-tissue mass in chest wall) may be the only feature differentiating mesothelioma from benign disease on CXR or CT.

Asbestosis

This is the term for the interstitial fibro-sis that develops in approximately 50% of patients with industrial asbestos exposure.

Interstitial change is best shown by HRCT and is an important factor in compensation assessment.

Interstitial fibrosis

Patients with interstitial fibrosis commonly present with dyspnoea, a dry

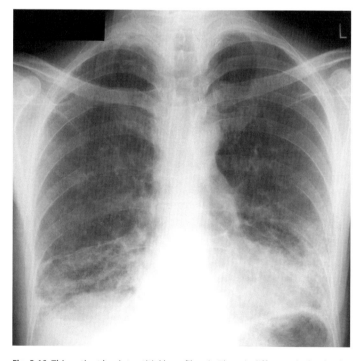

Fig. 3.16 This patient has interstitial lung fibrosis. There is diffuse reticular density in both lower zones with associated volume loss. The left heart border is ill-defined with a 'shaggy' appearance.

cough and restrictive pulmonary function tests. Causes include the following:

- Idiopathic
- It may be associated with other systemic conditions such as collagen vascular diseases, especially scleroderma and rheumatoid arthritis
- Asbestosis
- Sarcoidosis: fibrosis tends to occur in upper zones
- Chronic hypersensitivity pneumonitis: fibrosis tends to occur in upper zones
- Drug-induced fibrosis.

CXR (Fig. 3.16)

CXR may be normal in early disease (2–8%). Characteristic features include irregular lines giving a reticular pattern, progressing to characteristic basal peripheral ring shadowing (honeycomb lung). Septal lines and decreased lung volume may occur. A 'shaggy' heart border as a result of reticulation or ring shadows in the adjacent lung may be seen.

CT

HRCT is far more sensitive than the CXR for demonstrating interstitial fibrosis. The characteristic features on HRCT are peripheral ring shadows, subpleural lines, traction bronchiectasis and a 'ground glass' appearance. If there is 'ground glass' density that does not contain areas of bronchiectasis, then the changes may be reversed by steroid therapy. Linear changes suggest irreversible fibrosis.

Further reading

Armstong P, Wilson A, Dee P, Hansell DM, eds. *Imaging of Diseases of the Chest*. London: Harcourt, 2000.

Chapter 4: **Cardiovascular system**

This chapter covers:
Common conditions
- Cardiac failure
- Pulmonary embolism
- Deep venous thrombosis
- Aortic disease (including thoracic dissection, aneurysm rupture)
- Peripheral vascular disease
- Pericardial effusion, superior vena cava obstruction

Common presentations in which imaging can help
- Acute chest pain: cardiac ischaemia, pulmonary embolism, aortic dissection
- Acute shortness of breath: cardiac failure, pulmonary oedema
- Chronic chest pain: cardiac ischaemia, pericardial effusion

Imaging strategy

The CXR remains the mainstay of initial imaging assessment of these acute symptoms and can provide important diagnostic information:
- Cardiac silhouette and size
- Mediastinal/hilar contour
- Lungs for evidence of interstitial or air-space oedema in particular
- Pleural spaces: are pleural effusions present?

However, the amount of information that can be gleaned from a CXR in the acute situation may be limited. Elderly or confused patients may not be able to cooperate, resulting in rotated or poorly exposed radiographs. In acutely ill patients, radiographs need to be taken AP rather than PA. In AP films, the cassette is often wedged behind the patient, who is propped up in bed, and this means that the heart is some distance from the film, causing relative enlargement of the cardiac silhouette because of magnification. Therefore heart size cannot be reliably assessed on an AP film.

An estimate of heart size can be made on PA films—the cardiothoracic ratio (CTR). This represents transverse measurement of the heart at its widest point divided by the thoracic width at its widest point (measured from the inner rib margin, and should be <50% in adults).

Once a patient has been assessed and an initial working diagnosis formulated, further imaging is often required:
- US: arterial or venous colour Doppler ultrasound
- CT/CT angiography
- MR/MRA
- Conventional peripheral angiography
- NM.

These modalities are available in most radiology departments and can be accessed following discussion with a radiologist.

Most radiology departments will have protocols for investigation of certain conditions (e.g. pulmonary embolism) and it is useful to be aware of these. Ask for advice if you are not sure.

Certain cardiac investigations (e.g. echocardiography and cardiac angiography) are now routinely performed by cardiologists and are not covered in this chapter.

Cardiac failure

Cardiac failure commonly presents acutely, often in association with myocardial infarction, or as acute decompensation of chronic cardiac impairment, perhaps precipitated by sepsis (e.g. chest infection), particularly in the elderly.

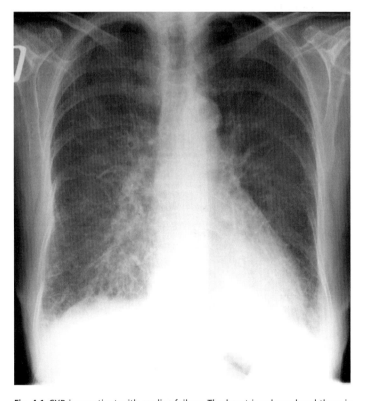

Fig. 4.1 CXR in a patient with cardiac failure. The heart is enlarged and there is evidence of widespread interstitial oedma with septal lines present. Septal lines are caused by interstitial oedema in interlobular lymphatics and are best seen as horizontal subpleural lines at the lung bases.

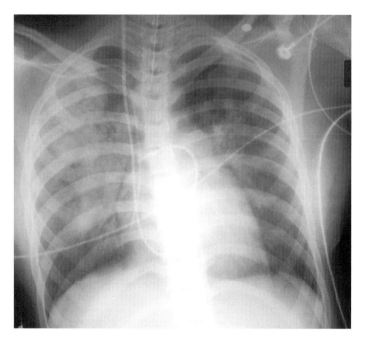

Fig. 4.2 CXR demonstrating diffuse alveolar (air-space) oedema in a young patient following intravenous fluid overload. The patient is intubated with a Swan–Ganz catheter and monitor leads are present.

CXR

The CXR is the mainstay of initial assessment. Look for:
• Cardiac enlargement (however, many films AP)
• Pleural effusion
• Pulmonary oedema. This may be interstitial (Fig. 4.1—look for septal lines, these are caused by interstitial oedema in the interlobular lymphatics) and fluid may spill over into the alveolar

air spaces to cause more confluent opacification (Fig. 4.2).

In pulmonary oedema, changes may be apparent on the CXR before the patient has symptoms, and conversely CXR abnormalities may persist when the patient is clinically well. Pulmonary oedema may be cardiogenic or non-cardiogenic (e.g. fluid overload, near drowning, smoke inhalation, fat embolism). In non-cardiogenic causes, the heart size may be normal (Fig. 4.2). Remember also that pulmonary oedema can appear unilateral on CXR if the patient has been lying on one side for some time prior to the radiograph being taken.

Pulmonary embolism

Pulmonary embolism (PE) represents a significant cause of mortality, particularly in the postoperative period (7–10 days post-procedure is the time of highest risk).

Patients present with shortness of breath, pleuritic chest pain and haemoptysis. Thrombus tends to originate within the deep veins of the lower limb, breaks off and embolizes to the lung. Pelvic veins are another common source of thrombus.

There is a wide spectrum of disease, ranging from recurrent small emboli over a prolonged period, which may result in pulmonary hypertension, to sudden death from massive embolism.

Most departments will have a protocol for imaging in acute PE.

CXR

- Frequently normal
- Atelectasis and/or consolidation may occur
- Arterial widening at the hilum resulting from embolus may be visible.

Lung scintigraphy (V/Q scan)

Involves performance of a ventilation and then a perfusion study with administration of inhaled and intravenously injected isotope (often ^{99m}Tc-based).

Examinations are reported as low, medium or high probability of PE, according to set criteria including CXR findings (Fig. 4.3a,b).

However, V/Q accuracy is reduced in several conditions (e.g. acute asthma, chronic obstructive airways disease or lung fibrosis) or where there is significant abnormality on the CXR with vascular redistribution.

Remember also that in many departments there is no routine NM service out of hours and also that isotope may need to be ordered from an off-site source.

CT

CT pulmonary angiography is a highly accurate technique that is being increasingly used to investigate suspected PE (Fig. 4.4). It can supplement intermediate probability V/Q scans if there is clinical concern and is helpful in those patients with abnormal CXRs where V/Q accuracy will be reduced.

Pulmonary angiography

With the advent of CT pulmonary angiography this technique is now used much less. It may still be helpful in difficult cases and also can be used to deliver thrombolysis directly into clot in patients with acute massive PE.

Colour Doppler US

This may be used to assess the lower limb leg veins in patients with suspected PE occult to imaging. Pelvic vein thrombus is often difficult to identify.

Lower limb deep venous thrombosis

Patients present with:

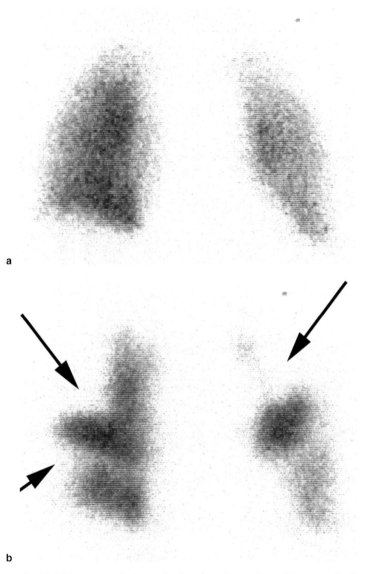

Fig. 4.3 (a) Normal ventilation study of the lungs in a patient with suspected pulmonary embolism. (b) Perfusion study in the same patient demonstrates multiple defects (areas of mismatch) consistent with emboli (arrows).

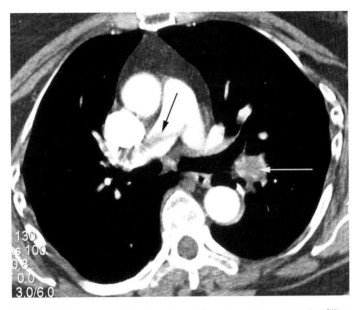

Fig. 4.4 Axial post-contrast CT demonstrates thrombus as low attenuation filling defect within enhancing right (black arrow) and left (white arrow) pulmonary arteries.

- Pain
- Swelling
- Positive Homan's sign (calf pain with foot dorsiflexion).

However, clinical examination is notoriously unreliable.

Risk factors for deep venous thrombosis (DVT) include:

- Surgery, especially on legs or pelvis
- Prolonged immobilization
- Malignancy
- Obesity
- Pregnancy or oral contraceptive pill.

Calf vein thrombus may propagate to involve the popliteal and/or femoral veins and it is at this stage that there is increased risk of PE.

Radiology departments will have management algorithms for the investigation of suspected lower limb DVT, following clinical DVT risk assessment.

US

US represents the initial imaging modality of choice.

Venous US is combined with D–dimer estimation in some centres. D–dimer is produced by the action of plasma on cross-linked fibrin and raised levels

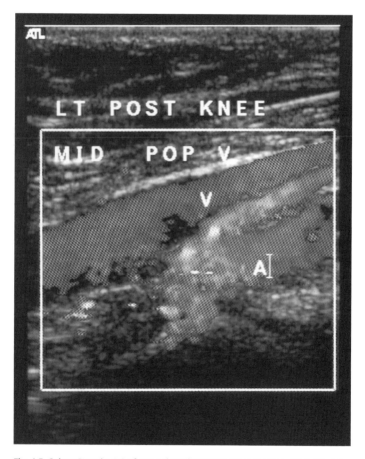

Fig. 4.5 Colour Doppler US of normal popliteal vein (V) and artery (A) behind the knee. Note normal flow in both vessels.

may be found in venous thromboembolic disorders. D-dimer can be used in combination with clinical assessment to establish which patients need imaging. Check protocols where you work.

The main sonographic features of venous thrombosis include identification of luminal thrombus, inability to compress the vein because of presence of thrombus, and absent or altered colour flow within the veins (Figs 4.5 & 4.6).

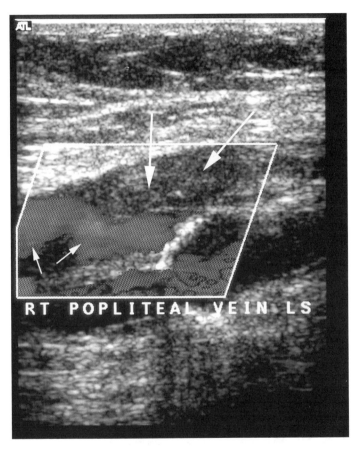

Fig. 4.6 Colour Doppler US in the same patient as Fig. 4.5 demonstrating popliteal thrombus (large white arrows) in the popliteal vein, with some colour flow seen in the vein above this (small white arrows).

US is accurate at demonstrating the deep veins in most patients but does have areas of weakness:

• Patients with fat or oedematous legs, or with extensive bandaging

• The vein can be difficult to visualize at the level of the adductor canal

• In patients who have had previous DVT, with subsequent venous deformity or scarring.

Usually, deep veins can be visualized down to the knee and one option that can be used if calf veins are initially poorly seen is to repeat the US at 7–10 days, if there is persisting clinical concern, to look for propagating thrombus.

Contrast X-ray venography

This is now little used because of the following:

- Invasive (needle in foot vein)
- Injection of iodinated contrast
- Use of ionizing radiation.

It has been largely replaced by US, but does have a role in technically difficult cases and post-phlebitic limbs.

Thoracic aortic dissection

Aortic dissection is caused by spontaneous separation of the aortic intima and adventitia by circulating blood having gained access to the media of the aortic wall, usually secondary to an intimal tear. Patients present with a sharp, tearing chest pain, often radiating to between the scapulae, and a heart murmur (from aortic regurgitation), asymmetric or absent peripheral pulses; shock or pleural effusion may also be present.

Hypertension is the most common cause, with Marfan's syndrome the other main aetiology.

CXR

CXR is usually performed initially and can be helpful. Mediastinal widening and cardiac enlargement (haemopericardium) may be present, but these areas are often difficult to assess on AP films. Further imaging should be arranged following discussion with radiologists and cardiologists. A combination of CT and echocardiography is often used initially.

CT

CT is accurate, as long as patients are stable and able to cooperate with breath-holding, in the identification of an intimal flap (Fig. 4.7) separating the two aortic channels (the true and false lumens) and also dissection extent.

The Stanford classification is easiest to remember:

- *Type A:* dissection involves ascending aorta with or without arch and needs surgical repair.
- *Type B:* dissection involves descending aorta distal to the left subclavian artery and may respond to medical treatment only.

CT may be degraded by streak artefacts from cardiac motion.

Transoesophageal echocardiography

This is a highly accurate adjunct for assessment of the ascending aorta.

MRI

This is used in some centres but is not widely available and problems can arise with patient monitoring during the procedure.

Aortography

This is accurate but invasive and may be performed following referral to a cardio-thoracic centre. In medically unfit patients, some centres use covered stents

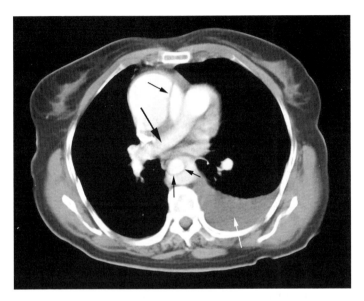

Fig. 4.7 Axial post-contrast CT in a patient with a type A thoracic aortic dissection. Intimal flaps are seen within the ascending (single small black arrow) and descending (paired small black arrows) thoracic aorta. Note normal pulmonary artery trunk (large black arrow) and a pleural effusion is present on the left (small white arrow).

deployed within the thoracic aortic true lumen to occlude the intimal tear and false lumen.

Abdominal aortic aneurysm

These are most commonly atherosclerotic in origin and are usually infrarenal, with iliac artery extension common.

Aneurysms may be asymptomatic and detected during routine clinical examination or during ultrasound examination of the abdomen. Patients with aneurysms may present with an abdominal mass or with pain. Patients with aneurysm leak or rupture present with pain, often radiating to the back with hypotension and an often palpable and tender mass.

The risk of aneurysm leak or rupture increases with increasing aneurysm size. Ruptured aortic aneurysm has a high mortality. Aortic size >3 cm on ultrasound represents aneurysmal dilatation. Aneurysms >5 cm in diameter should be considered for surgical repair, although in some centres aneurysms may be considered for stent grafting, especially in medically unfit patients.

If you have any suspicion that you are dealing with a leaking aneurysm, contact senior surgical and anaesthetic colleagues urgently.

Haemodynamically unstable patients need to be transferred to theatre. If patients are stable, or if the diagnosis is in doubt, imaging may be indicated.

AXR

This is often performed as part of abdominal pain assessment. Calcification in an aneurysmal aorta may be apparent. If there has been retroperitoneal haemorrhage, a mass may be present with enlargement or loss of psoas outline.

US

US can be useful for identification of an aneurysm, but access to the retroperitoneum is often limited.

CT

CT is the modality of choice for the diagnosis of suspected aneurysm leak in stable patients (Fig. 4.8) and also for aneurysm assessment prior to surgery in elective aneurysm repairs. CT will demonstrate aneurysm extent and its relation to the renal and common iliac arteries.

Peripheral vascular disease

There are a number of modalities now available for evaluation of the lower limb arterial supply in patients presenting with symptoms of claudication, rest pain or acute ischaemia.

Colour Doppler US and MRA represent non-invasive and accurate means of mapping out the arterial supply of the lower limbs in patients with chronic symptoms.

Conventional X-ray angiography may be performed in patients with suspected stenoses identified with US or MRA prior to therapeutic intervention or in patients with acute ischaemia, perhaps secondary to an embolus.

Angiography is usually performed via a femoral artery puncture, with a catheter introduced into the lower abdominal aorta and contrast injected. If a stenosis or occlusion is identified, this may be treated via angioplasty (balloon dilatation) or insertion of a metallic stent (Figs 4.9 & 4.10).

Patient preparation for angiography

• Consent: this may be obtained by a senior surgical colleague or radiologist. Check the protocol.
• IV cannula insertion.
• Check full blood count and clotting profile.
• Bleeding diathesis is a contraindication and you always need to inform the radiologist if the patient is taking warfarin.
• If the patient is on metformin, this should be stopped the day before the procedure.
• The patient should be fasted for 4 hr before the procedure.

Complications of angiography

At puncture site:
• Thrombosis or occlusion
• Haematoma

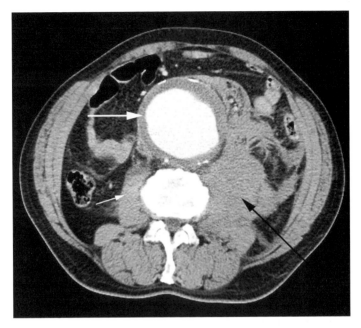

Fig. 4.8 Axial post-contrast CT in a patient with a leaking aortic aneurysm. The aorta is aneurysmal (large white arrow) and there is extensive retroperitoneal haemorrhage on the left (black arrow). Note normal right psoas muscle (small white arrow).

- Pseudoaneurysm
- Infection
- Nerve damage
- Arteriovenous fistula.

Patients with acute limb ischaemia with occluding thrombus demonstrated angiographically may be suitable for thrombolysis. Using this technique, a catheter is manipulated near to the thrombus and a thrombolytic agent infused directly (e.g. recombinant tissue plasminogen activator; rtPA).

There are several contraindications to the use of thrombolysis:
- Active internal bleeding
- Recent cerebrovascular accident (within 6 months) including transient ischaemic attack (TIA) (within 2 months)
- Intracranial tumour
- Recent major surgery, organ biopsy or trauma
- Uncontrolled hypertension
- Known active peptic ulceration

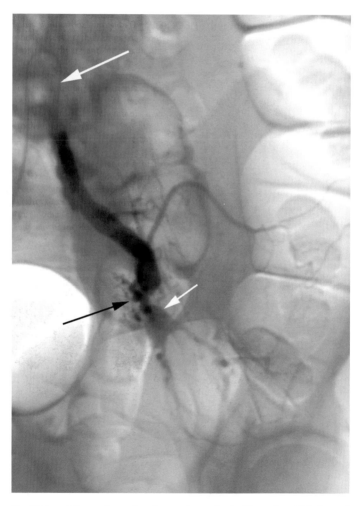

Fig. 4.9 Image from a femoral angiogram in a patient with an absent left femoral pulse and left leg pain. The catheter has been passed up the right femoral artery and over the aortic bifurcation (large white arrow) and contrast injected. This demonstrates occlusion of the left external iliac artery (black arrow) with some contrast in the left internal iliac artery, which also appears occluded soon after its origin (small white arrow).

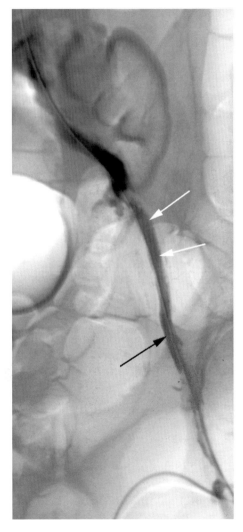

Fig. 4.10 Image from the same patient as Fig. 4.9, demonstrating a metallic stent deployed over a catheter traversing the external iliac occlusion (white arrows) with contrast passing distally (black arrow), confirming vessel patency.

• Proliferative diabetic retinopathy or history of vitreous haemorrhage.

Patients must be carefully monitored during thrombolytic administration for evidence of haemorrhage and repeat angiography will be required to demonstrate vessel patency. Keep in close contact with the radiologist involved.

Pericardial effusion

Pericardial effusion may occur in:
• Cardiac or renal failure
• Post-trauma
• Post-myocardial infarction or aortic dissection
• Post-infective (e.g. viral, TB).

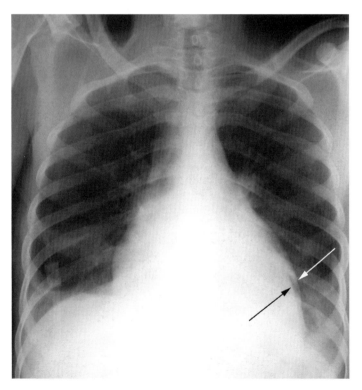

Fig. 4.11 CXR in a patient with tuberculous pericardial effusion. The heart is enlarged and lucency is well demonstrated (between arrows) at the left heart border, resulting from pericardial fluid.

CXR

This represents the usual initial imaging modality. Look for:
• Globally enlarged cardiac silhouette
• Rapidly appearing cardiomegaly on serial CXRs, with normal pulmonary vascularity
• An increase in lucency at the heart margin, brought about by difference in density of the heart muscle and adjacent pericardial fluid (Fig. 4.11).

Echocardiography

This will confirm the presence of effu-sion and can be used to guide therapeutic or diagnostic aspiration.

Superior vena cava syndrome

This is caused by superior vena cava obstruction (SVCO) with develop-ment of collateral pathways and is usually secondary to compression via mediastinal bronchial carcinoma or lymphoma.

Patients present with head or neck oedema, headaches and cutaneous venous collateral channels.

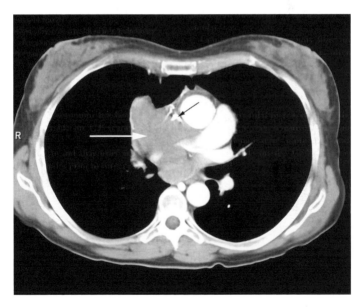

Fig. 4.12 Post-contrast CT in a patient with superior vena cava (SVC) obstruction caused by squamous cell lung carcinoma. A large mass is present (white arrow) markedly compressing the SVC (black arrow).

CXR

This may demonstrate a mediastinal mass. Look for evidence of mediastinal adenopathy, bony and lung metastases.

CT

CT is the next investigation of choice. It will delineate the superior vena cava (SVC) with the level of compression and demonstrate a mediastinal mass (Fig. 4.12). Metastases to bone, lungs and liver can also be demonstrated, together with SVC thrombus.

SVC venography

This may be useful in some cases. It is performed following injection of contrast into an arm vein and delineates the level and extent of compression and the presence of associated or causative thrombus. Some patients may be suitable for insertion of an SVC stent across a stricture for palliative purposes to relieve obstruction.

Further reading

Hagspiel KD, Matsumoto AH, eds. *Radiologic Clinics of North America: Vascular Imaging*; 2002; Volume 40 (4).

Chapter 5: **The upper gastrointestinal tract**

This chapter covers:
Common conditions
• Oesophagus: carcinoma, oesophagitis and peptic stricture, achalasia
• Stomach: carcinoma
• Small bowel: obstruction, pneumoperitoneum, Crohn's disease, malabsorption
• Also, leiomyoma, gastric volvulus, gastric dilatation
Common presentations in which imaging can help
• Dysphagia: peptic stricture, carcinoma of oesophagus or stomach, oesophagitis
• Haematemesis: ulceration, carcinoma, varices
• Dyspepsia: ulceration, gastritis
• Acute abdominal pain: obstruction, pancreatitis, perforation
• Weight loss or anaemia with any of the above: particularly carcinoma, ulceration
• Many symptoms relating to the upper gastrointestinal tract are now investigated primarily with endoscopy, with barium studies reserved for patients who are unfit or who decline endoscopy

Imaging strategy

Endoscopy

Endoscopy is the main investigation for abnormalities of the upper gastrointestinal (GI) tract, although barium studies are useful in those patients who are unfit or decline endoscopy. Endoscopy has the benefit of easy biopsy of any lesions seen.

Barium examination

This remains the initial modality of choice for dysphagia in many centres and is also the primary investigation for suspected small bowel pathology.

Identifying the most likely site of pathology in the request is important (e.g. oesophagus, stomach or small bowel), so that the patient can be prepared for a barium swallow, meal or small bowel follow-through. In addition, it guides the radiologist to select the best barium preparation. Different barium suspensions are used for each area to maximize coating and diagnostic accuracy.

If a small bowel enema is required it is often helpful to discuss this with a radiologist as there are different ways of conducting the examination that require particular preparation of the patient.

For patients with suspected acute perforation or bowel obstruction, a supine AXR and erect CXR should be requested. Other things to look for on the CXR are metastases in oesophageal or gastric carcinoma, or aspiration pneumonia and oesophageal dilatation in achalasia and carcinoma.

CT

CT is the technique of choice for staging upper gastrointestinal tract malignancy and is being increasingly used.

MR, US and NM

These do not have prominent roles in primary investigation of upper gastrointestinal tract disease. Interventional radiology does have techniques to offer in palliative treatment of mechanical obstruction.

Oesophageal carcinoma

The majority of oesophageal carcinomas are squamous cell in origin, although adenocarcinoma arising within columnar-lined epithelium (Barrett's oesophagus) is an increasingly recognized subgroup.

Most patients with oesophageal carcinoma present with dysphagia, and barium swallow is frequently performed as the initial imaging investigation.

Barium swallow

Early carcinomas appear as small sessile polyps or plaques. Some lesions appear as superficial spreading lesions, giving irregularity and nodularity of the mucosa (Fig. 5.1).

Advanced carcinomas appear as large, polypoidal, often ulcerating lesions and have features of luminal stricturing with shouldering and an 'apple core' appearance (Fig. 5.2).

Patients with suspected oesophageal carcinoma on barium examination will proceed to endoscopy for histological confirmation and will undergo further imaging if they are considered suitable for further treatment.

CXR

Many patients have a CXR at the time of initial barium examination and a dilated oesophagus may be apparent occasionally. Also look for evidence of aspiration, pneumonia and lung and rib metastases.

CT

This is currently the best, relatively non-invasive test for staging oesophageal carcinoma and identifying features of inoperability which include:
• Invasion of local structures (e.g. aorta, pericardium, diaphragm)
• Associated adenopathy
• Metastases to lung or liver.

MR

This is currently less accurate than CT.

Endoscopic US

This is accurate and complementary to CT in assessing local extent of tumour and local nodal status.

PET

A major problem for CT is detecting tumour in normal-sized nodes (nodal enlargement is the main CT criterion for malignancy). PET has been shown to be effective at detecting nodal metastases occult on CT.

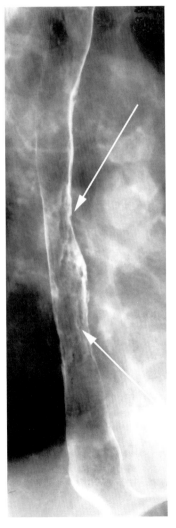

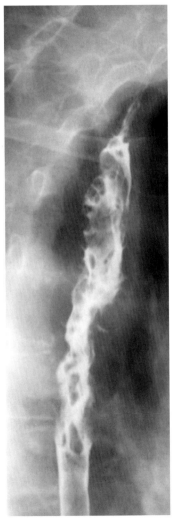

Fig. 5.1 Film from barium swallow demonstrates a superficial spreading oesophageal carcinoma (arrows). Note nodularity and irregularity of mucosa.

Fig. 5.2 Advanced oesophageal carcinoma on barium swallow. There is a large polypoidal mass with stricturing, mucosal irregularity and ulceration.

Palliative treatment

Many patients turn out to be inoperable or unfit for radical surgery. Dysphagia is frequently a problem and can be palliated with radiological insertion of a metallic stent over a guidewire to cross and then dilate the tumour.

Oesophagitis

Reflux oesophagitis and peptic stricture

Most patients who present with symptoms of gastro-oesophageal reflux and reflux oesophagitis will undergo endoscopic assessment if conventional drug treatments fail.

Persistent reflux oesophagitis may initiate the development of a peptic stricture, usually manifested by slowly progressive dysphagia. Barium studies are useful for initial assessment in such patients.

Most peptic strictures are in the distal oesophagus and they appear smooth and tapered on barium examination (Fig. 5.3). These lesions should always be assessed endoscopically to exclude malignancy and can be considered for balloon dilatation.

Infective oesophagitis

Candidiasis is the most common cause of infective oesophagitis, although herpes simplex and cytomegalovirus may also be responsible. *Candida* infection usually occurs in the immunocompromised patient and spreads down from the mouth.

Patients often present with severe and painful dysphagia, and barium swallow is used to confirm the diagnosis.

Candida oesophagitis appears as discrete plaque-like lesions that are mucosal and occur in the upper and mid-oesophagus (Fig. 5.4). Plaques may coalesce to give a 'shaggy' appearance.

Achalasia of the oesophagus

Achalasia is caused by a failure of normal peristalsis and relaxation at the level of the lower oesophageal sphincter. The cause is unknown but it may be neurogenic in origin. Patients tend to be middle-aged and present with slowly progressive dysphagia. Regurgitation of food contents and aspiration may occur.

There is an increased risk of oesophageal carcinoma in achalasia.

Request barium swallow and CXR initially. Barium swallow demonstrates oesophageal dilatation, which may be massive and contain significant food residue. Normal peristalsis is absent and typically the lower oesophagus has a narrowed 'beak-like' appearance (Fig. 5.5).

The dilated oesophagus may be visible on CXR, often in the right paratracheal region and the normal stomach bubble is absent. An air–fluid level may be seen as high as the manubrium.

Endoscopy should also be performed to exclude malignancy (food residue can make this difficult).

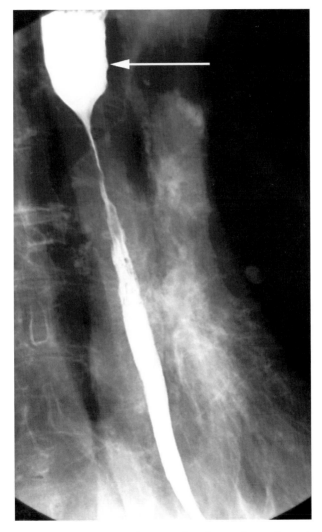

Fig. 5.3 Peptic-type stricture in the upper thoracic oesophagus demonstrated on barium swallow. Note tapered appearance and smooth margins. The upper oesophagus is dilated (arrow).

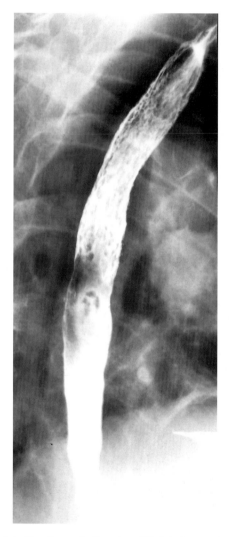

Fig. 5.4 Barium swallow demonstration of candidiasis in the oesophagus. Multiple mucosal plaques are present. Oral *Candida* is usually present, allowing correct diagnosis, and the disease responds promptly to antifungal treatment.

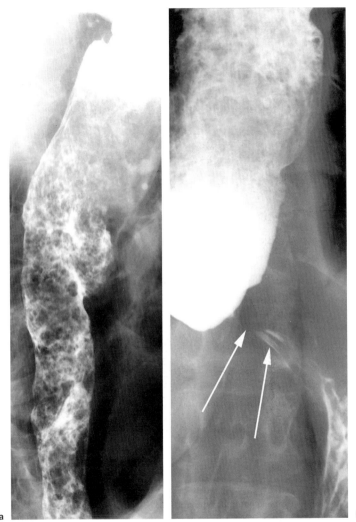

a   b

Fig. 5.5 (a,b) Two films from a barium swallow series in a patient with achalasia. There is gross dilatation of the oesophagus, which contains food residue and smooth narrowing of the lumen is seen in the distal oesophagus (arrows in b).

Gastric carcinoma

Patients present with vague symptoms, including epigastric discomfort, anorexia and weight loss. Most gastric carcinomas are adenocarcinomas and tend to be advanced at the time of diagnosis. Prognosis is poor.

AXR

AXR may show gastric mass or calcification in tumour or metastases. Calcification is rare, but may occur in mucin-producing scirrhous carcinomas.

Gastric outflow obstruction may be evident with antral tumours.

CXR

Look for lung metastases and pleural effusion.

Barium meal

This used to be the mainstay of diagnosis of gastric carcinoma but has been largely replaced by endoscopy. Barium meal may still be useful in some circumstances:
• Scirrhous carcinoma may extend

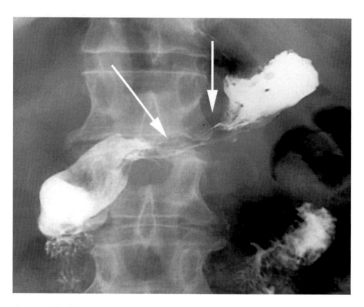

Fig. 5.6 Film from barium meal examination in a patient with gastric carcinoma and 'leather-bottle' gastric configuration. Note diffuse narrowing of stomach body (arrows).

extensively and submucosally in the stomach giving a 'leather-bottle' appearance (Fig. 5.6). Occasionally, the stomach mucosa may look normal endoscopically and deeper biopsies are required.

• Barium can be used to assess the extent of a gastric carcinoma if palliative insertion of expanding metallic stents is being considered.

CT

CT is the imaging modality of choice for staging gastric carcinoma (Fig. 5.7). CT will:

• Demonstrate a gastric mass or wall thickening
• Confirm stage of tumour and operability by demonstrating:
  – Invasion of local structures
  – Metastases along peritoneal ligaments with mesenteric nodal involvement and ascites
  – Involvement of regional lymph nodes
  – Liver, lung and ovarian metastases.

Endoscopic US

This can be used as a complementary modality to CT for assessing tumour ex-

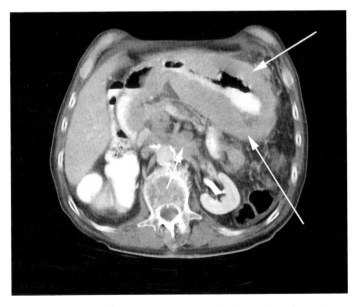

Fig. 5.7 Post-contrast CT in a patient with locally advanced gastric carcinoma. There is diffuse thickening of the stomach wall (long arrows) and bulky left gastric and coeliac adenopathy is present (short arrow).

tension into the gastric wall and involvement of local lymph nodes.

Leiomyoma

More than 50% of all benign oesophageal tumours are leiomyomas, which comprise encapsulated bands of smooth muscle and fibrous tissue.

Gastric leiomyoma is the second most common benign stomach tumour and leiomyomas also are common in the small bowel. Gastric leiomyoma appears as a submucosal mass on barium examination and CT and may ulcerate.

Oesophageal leiomyoma is often asymptomatic, although patients may present with dysphagia or haematemesis. Masses can be seen on CXR when large calcification is a feature. These tumours appear as smooth submucosal lesions on barium swallow (Fig. 5.8).

Leiomyomas are at risk of malignant sarcomatous degeneration.

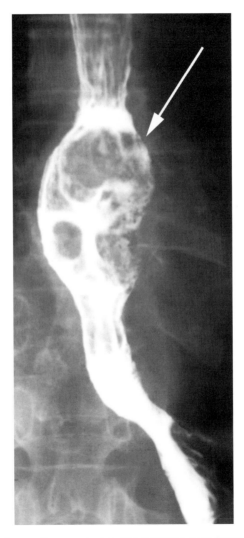

Fig. 5.8 Barium swallow examination demonstrates a large leiomyoma in the lower oesophagus (arrow).

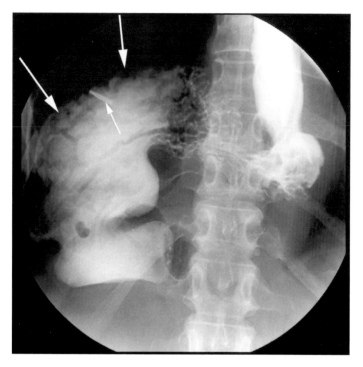

Fig. 5.9 Barium meal examination demonstrates organo-axial volvulus of the stomach with the stomach intrathoracic and greater curve (long arrows) above the lesser curve. Note tip of nasogastric tube (short arrow).

Gastric volvulus

This is an uncommon acquired twist of the stomach that may cause outflow obstruction. It is caused by abnormal stomach suspensory ligaments and often elongated gastrocolic and gastrohepatic mesenteries allowing stomach rotation.

A diaphragmatic defect (e.g. hernia or eventration) is often also present.

In organo–axial volvulus, the stomach rotates upward around a line extending from cardia to pylorus (long axis) (Fig. 5.9). In mesentero–axial volvulus, the stomach rotates around a line from lesser to greater curvature.

Patients present with pain, inability to

vomit and there is also difficulty passing a nasogastric tube or barium into the stomach.

An erect CXR may demonstrate an air–fluid level in the chest. Barium studies may show stomach inversion with greater curve above the lesser curve (Fig. 5.9).

Complications include gastric outflow obstruction, with dilatation and perforation.

Gastric dilatation

Gastric dilatation with outflow obstruction

Peptic ulcer disease is the most common cause. Other important causes include carcinoma of the stomach or duodenal invasion by pancreatic carcinoma.

AXR

AXR demonstrates the outline of a dilated gas-filled stomach that may contain food residue. Look for air in the stomach wall secondary to ischaemia.

Patients often proceed to a barium study in the first instance, where a cause may be identified (Fig. 5.10). Alternatively, a nasogastric tube can be passed and the stomach emptied and then endoscopy attempted.

Gastric dilatation without outflow obstruction

Acute gastric retention can occur without mechanical obstruction, but this needs to be excluded.

Acute gastric dilatation can occur postoperatively and in other medical conditions (e.g. diabetes) and is characterized by acute severe distension of the stomach with gas and fluid. Vomiting and circulatory collapse may follow if diagnosis and treatment (nasogastric tube, correct electrolytes, rehydrate) is not prompt.

Small bowel obstruction

Adhesions following previous surgery are the most common cause of small bowel obstruction. Obstructed hernia, gallstone ileus, small bowel volvulus, tumour and stricture (e.g. Crohn's disease) should also be considered. The diagnosis of small bowel obstruction can usually be made following clinical examination and AXR. Patients present with pain, vomiting and constipation. On examination, high-pitched tinkling sounds are typical of a mechanical obstruction. Although the AXR findings in obstruction and ileus are similar, bowel sounds tend to be diminished in ileus.

AXR

Generally, AXR is performed supine and in small bowel obstruction will demonstrate multiple dilated loops of gas-filled small bowel. Small bowel tends to be centrally located in the abdomen. Valvulae conniventes are thin mucosal lines that traverse the whole bowel lumen, seen best in the proximal small bowel.

Sometimes, when dilated, small bowel loops are fluid-filled and it may be hard to identify these. Here an erect AXR may be helpful by demonstrating air–fluid levels in small bowel. Dilated small bowel loops may have a 'stepladder' appearance (Fig. 5.11) in low obstruction

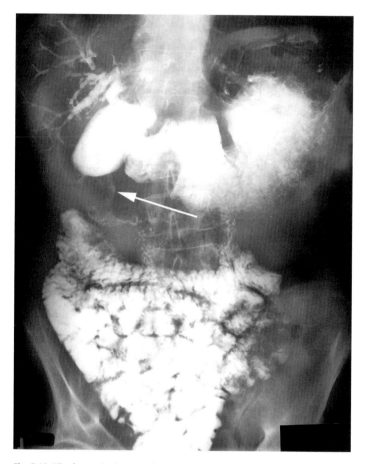

Fig. 5.10 Film from a barium meal examination at a delay with small bowel opacification also. There is stomach distension, with food residue seen in the stomach. Luminal narrowing and mucosal irregularity in the second part of the duodenum secondary to pancreatic malignancy (arrow) is responsible. Obstruction is not complete. Note barium reflux into biliary tree secondary to previous sphincterotomy.

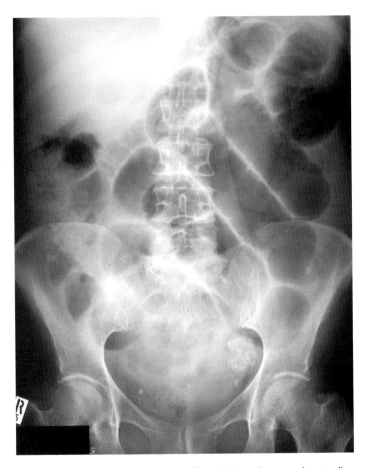

Fig. 5.11 Supine AXR in a patient with small bowel obstruction secondary to adhesions. The dilated small bowel loops are arranged in a 'stepladder' configuration. Note valvulae conniventes traversing bowel lumen.

(the greater the number of loops the lower the obstruction). Look for:

• Air in biliary tree and impacted gallstone in the distal ileum in gallstone ileus

• Air in obstructed femoral or inguinal hernia sac

• Evidence of perforation

• Sacroiliitis (Crohn's disease).

If there is no history of previous surgery and patients do not settle with conservative treatment, further imaging can be considered prior to laparotomy.

Barium follow-through or small bowel enema

Technically, results are often poor with dilution of barium and flocculation in obstructed bowel. If obstruction resolves, barium studies can then be performed electively and are often helpful.

US

This can differentiate small from large bowel but is rarely diagnostic of the cause of obstruction.

CT

This is often very useful in diagnosing the cause of small bowel obstruction and also in assessing small bowel ischaemia. No oral contrast is needed and extramural information is also acquired.

Pneumoperitoneum

There are a large number of causes of free air within the peritoneal cavity, but the cause most commonly seen as an emergency is that from a perforated viscus (e.g. gastric or duodenal ulcer, appendix, diverticulum, caecal volvulus or toxic megacolon). Iatrogenic causes should also be recognized (e.g. leaking surgical anastomosis, post-laparoscopy [air not normally seen after 3 days], endoscopic perforation). Post-laparotomy air can persist 'normally' for up to 10 days.

Suspected perforation of a viscus is usually imaged initially with a supine AXR and an erect CXR (allowing free intraperitoneal air to rise under the diaphragm). If there is persisting clinical concern and initial films are unhelpful, a left lateral decubitus radiograph may be diagnostic. The patient lies on the left side for 10–15 minutes and a horizontal beam radiograph is taken. As little as 1 ml of free air can be detected beneath the lateral liver and the abdominal wall.

Patterns of pneumoperitoneum on supine AXR

• Rigler's sign: free intraperitoneal air outlines the outside of the bowel wall with luminal gas outlining the inner aspect (Fig. 5.12).
• Gas may accumulate between the anterior aspect of the liver and the abdominal wall causing increased lucency in the right upper quadrant (Fig. 5.12).
• Air may track into Morison's pouch (an intraperitoneal recess between liver and right kidney).
• Air may outline peritoneal ligaments (e.g. falciform and ligamentum teres).

Pneumoperitoneum on erect CXR

An erect CXR is extremely sensitive in detecting small amounts of free intraperitoneal air (Figs 5.13 & 5.14). But do not be caught out—air within the gastric fundus can simulate air beneath the left hemidiaphragm, as can fat. Bowel can also intersperse between liver and right hemidiaphragm, mimicking free air (Chilaiditi's syndrome) (Fig. 5.15).

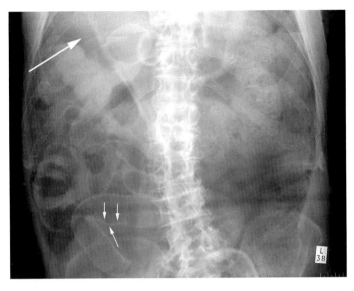

Fig. 5.12 Supine AXR in a patient with pneumoperitoneum secondary to appendix perforation. Rigler's sign is well demonstrated, with small bowel wall clearly outlined by luminal air within (paired small arrows) and free intraperitoneal air outside (single short arrow). Note also increased lucency in right upper quadrant (long arrow) resulting from free air between liver and abdominal wall.

Other imaging

CT is extremely sensitive at detecting small amounts of free intraperitoneal air (Fig. 5.16).

Occasionally, water-soluble contrast studies are used to identify sites of bowel perforation (remember barium is contraindicated in suspected perforation— it causes peritonitis).

Pneumoretroperitoneum

Retroperitoneal portions of the bowel (duodenum, ascending or descending colon, rectum) can also perforate. Air may be seen in relation to the psoas muscles or within the pararenal regions.

Crohn's disease

Crohn's disease is a chronic relapsing disease that can affect any part of the gastrointestinal tract from the mouth to the anus. Patients with the small bowel involved present with pain, diarrhoea and weight loss and often a right iliac fossa mass. The small bowel is involved in 80% of patients, with

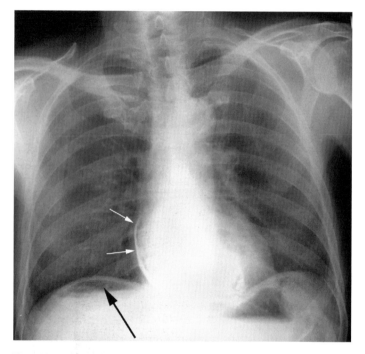

Fig. 5.13 Erect CXR demonstrating a small amount of subdiaphragmatic free intraperitoneal air (black arrow). Note pericardial calcification secondary to previous tuberculous pericarditis (short arrows).

the terminal ileum the most common location.

Small bowel barium follow-through or small bowel barium enema (enteroclysis) are the investigations of choice for suspected small bowel Crohn's disease, or for evaluation of disease extent or disease in relapse. Small bowel enema involves the passage of a feeding tube into the jejunum and then injection of diluted barium to opacify the small bowel. It is more accurate than small bowel follow-through, which involves drinking a barium solution, but has drawbacks. Patients often do not tolerate nasojejunal intubation and the procedure may be time-consuming with a high radiation dose. Many centres use small bowel follow-through initially.

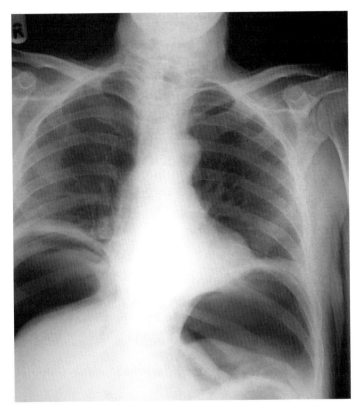

Fig. 5.14 Erect CXR with extensive subdiaphragmatic free air.

Barium features of small bowel Crohn's disease (Fig. 5.17)

Early
Small bowel fold thickening
Hyperplasia of lymphoid follicles with or without mucosal erosions (aphthous ulcer)
Aphthous ulcers enlarge and deepen transmurally — 'rose-thorn' ulcers

Late
Deep ulcers or fissures
Pseudopolyps
Transverse and longitudinal fissures may surround pseudopolyps — 'cobblestone' pattern
Separation of oedematous bowel loops

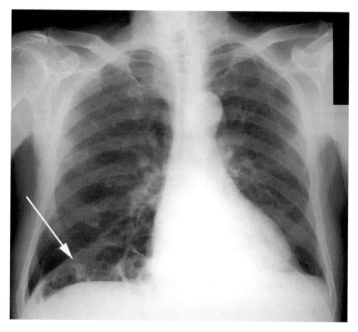

Fig. 5.15 Erect CXR in a patient with large bowel interposed between liver and right hemidiaphragm (arrow; Chilaiditi's syndrome). This can be confused with pneumoperitoneum.

Lesions often occur in multiple sites along the bowel, giving rise to the description of 'skip' lesions. Strictures are common, especially in the terminal ileum and these may cause obstruction, requiring surgical intervention.

Complications of small bowel Crohn's disease

• *Fistula formation:* in up to one-third of patients, with ileocaecal and entero-

enteric most common. These are usually well demonstrated on barium examination. Contrast can be inserted via a catheter placed into the fistula to demonstrate deep connections (fistulogram).
• *Abscess:* caused by local perforation and best demonstrated with CT (which can also be used to guide percutaneous drainage).
• *Adenocarcinoma:* increased incidence, especially at the site of chronic fistulation.

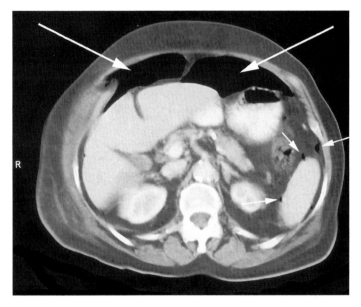

Fig. 5.16 Post-contrast CT in a patient with pneumoperitoneum following perforation of sigmoid diverticular disease. Free air is identified anterior to the liver (long arrows) and as small pockets within the upper abdomen (small arrows).

Malabsorption

Malabsorption can be caused by:
• Digestive enzyme deficiency (e.g. chronic pancreatitis, Crohn's terminal ileitis)
• Mucosal abnormality (e.g. coeliac disease, widespread Crohn's disease, Whipple's disease, short bowel syndrome)
• Secondary to bacterial overgrowth (e.g. diverticulosis, blind-loop syndrome).

Malabsorption can be difficult to diagnose. Clinical features include steatorrhoea, diarrhoea, weight loss and features of anaemia or vitamin deficiency. A range of haematological and biochemical tests are available but intestinal mucosal biopsy is frequently the diagnostic investigation.

Barium studies

Small bowel follow-through or small bowel enema (see above) are the imaging investigations commonly requested initially. A range of abnormalities may be demonstrated on barium studies, but

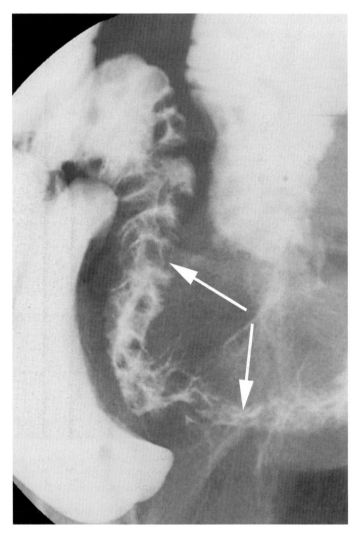

Fig. 5.17 Spot views of the terminal ileum in a patient with Crohn's disease. There is diffuse abnormality of the distal small bowel, which is narrowed, with irregular mucosa (arrows). Ulceration is present. Note separation of oedematous small bowel loops.

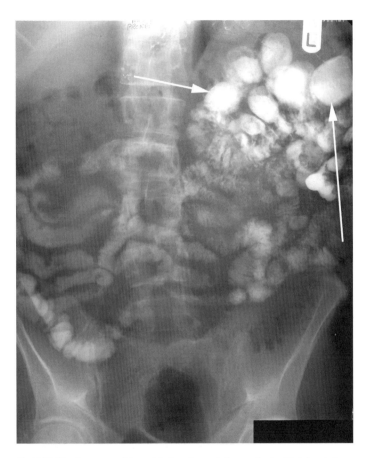

Fig. 5.18 Film from a small bowel follow-through in a patient with jejunal diverticulosis. Multiple diverticula are present in the jejunum (arrows); these cause malabsorption secondary to bacterial overgrowth in diverticula and may require surgery if medical management fails.

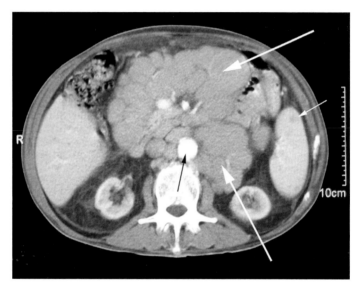

Fig. 5.19 Post-contrast CT in a patient with biopsy-proven lymphomatous infiltration of the small bowel. There is extensive mesenteric and para-aortic adenopathy in association (long arrows) and a lymphoma deposit is also seen in the spleen (short white arrow). The normal enhancing aorta is indicated (black arrow).

these are frequently non-specific. Look for regular or irregular mucosal fold thickening and small bowel dilatation.

Barium examination may reveal more specific causes (e.g. jejunal diverticulosis [Fig. 5.18], Crohn's disease).

CT and MR

CT and MR may be useful for further assessment of the small bowel wall and also of adjacent mesentery, lymph nodes, liver and spleen if systemic disorder (e.g. lymphoma) is suspected (Fig. 5.19).

Further reading

Gore RM, Levine MS, eds. *Textbook of Gastrointestinal Radiology*, 2nd edn. Philadelphia: Saunders, 2000.

Levine MS, Rubesin SE, Laufer I, eds. *Double Contrast Gastrointestinal Radiology*, 3rd edn. Philadelphia: Saunders, 2000.

Miller FH, ed. *The Radiological Clinics of North America: Radiology of the Pancreas, Gall bladder and Biliary Tract*, Vol. 40. 2002.

Chapter 6: **The lower gastrointestinal tract**

This chapter covers:
Common conditions
- Appendicitis
- Colonic obstruction
- Diverticular disease
- Neoplasia: polyp, carcinoma
- Sepsis
- Colitis
- Volvulus

Common presentations in which imaging can help
- Altered bowel habit: obstruction, carcinoma, diverticular disease
- Acute abdominal distension: obstruction
- Acute abdominal pain: obstruction, colitis, diverticulitis
- Rectal bleeding: carcinoma, diverticular disease, colitis

Look for hepatomegaly or an abdominal mass on clinical examination.

Patients should undergo perianal and rectal examination at presentation. This task is often delegated to the house officer. If you are unsure, ask for help from a senior colleague.

Imaging strategy

Initial imaging in acute presentations usually involves a supine AXR and an erect CXR. CXR may demonstrate free intraperitoneal air beneath the diaphragm (see Chapter 5), and many patients who are acutely ill may have evidence of chest sepsis or cardiac failure

also. Supine AXR will give information concerning small and large bowel gas pattern, free intraperitoneal air, soft tissues and bony structures.

Once initial clinical assessment has been made and a working diagnosis formulated, many patients will require further imaging. Discuss the case with the radiologist to identify the best way (including endoscopy) to reach a diagnosis.

US

US in colorectal disease can be helpful for initial assessment of:
- Possible bowel-related mass
- Free fluid or abscess formation
- Solid organs.

By their nature, many pathologies of the colon are associated with significant bowel gas and when combined with an elderly, immobile or obese patient the use of US may be limited.

CT

CT can provide significant additional diagnostic information in patients with bowel-related masses and suspected inflammatory disease or malignancy. CT is increasingly being used as an early investigation in the elderly and frail to avoid rectal contrast studies.

Contrast enema

This is an essential tool for evaluation of

the rectum and colon (combined with endoscopy).

Unprepared contrast enema, usually using water-soluble iodinated contrast, may be used to exclude an obstructing lesion in patients with large bowel obstruction. Mucosal detail is poor and, if the study is negative, follow-up barium enema or colonoscopy is often needed.

Contrast enema should not be performed in patients at risk of perforation (e.g. toxic megacolon). Barium causes peritonitis if it extravasates outside the bowel and should not be used in patients who may have perforation or where recent deep biopsies have been performed. Water-soluble contrast should be used.

Maximum diagnostic information is obtained using the double-contrast technique (air and barium) with good bowel preparation. However, a significant number of elderly patients cannot retain air and/or barium and may be immobile. In some of these patients, CT may be used to exclude a gross mass lesion.

MR

MR has a role in staging colorectal carcinoma, but its use is currently limited otherwise.

NM

This has a limited role, but it can be used to assess the extent of inflammatory colitis.

Appendicitis

This is the most common surgical emergency, with a peak incidence in the second and third decades.

The classic signs of appendicitis are absent in up to one-third of patients and there is a significant rate of clinical misdiagnosis.

Imaging may be particularly helpful in:
• The elderly, where symptoms and signs may be minimal
• Children, where history and examination are often difficult
• Young women who may have a gynaecological cause for pain.

Accurate and appropriate imaging reduces the number of normal laparotomies and will help to exclude other causes of appendix-type pain. However, imaging is often not needed following clinical assessment.

AXR

Look for:
• Laminated calcified appendicolith (10–15% of patients)
• Evidence of ileus, often localized to the right iliac fossa
• Distortion of psoas margin
• Bubbles of air in associated appendix abscess.

US

This represents a non-invasive modality for assessment of atypical patients. US is most accurate in children and young and/or pregnant women, where the appendix is not obscured by gas. US features of appendicitis include identification of the appendix as an abnormal, thick-walled and non-compressible structure with a distended lumen (Fig. 6.1). An appendicolith or associated abscess formation may also be seen.

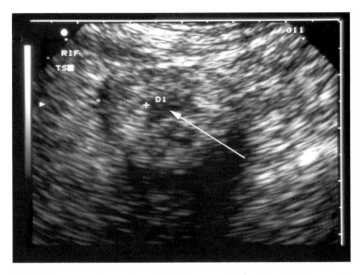

Fig. 6.1 Transverse ultrasound section of the appendix in a patient with appendicitis. The appendix has a thickened wall (callipers) with a dilated lumen (arrow) and a target appearance.

CT

CT is highly accurate in the evaluation of appendix inflammation and local extent. It is the technique of choice in the elderly, obese or very tender patients or where US has been unhelpful and clinical concern persists.

Barium studies

Barium studies of small or large bowel may be helpful in some patients where initial US or CT have indicated bowel pathology not clearly related to the appendix.

Colonic obstruction

The major causes of large bowel obstruction are carcinoma, diverticular disease and volvulus. Carcinoma, most commonly within the sigmoid, accounts for > 50% of cases. Symptoms are of abdominal distension and pain with associated vomiting. A mass may be palpable.

The integrity of the ileocaecal valve is important. If it is competent, this prevents passage of air into the small bowel if the large bowel is obstructed, leading to rapid and pronounced colonic and caecal dilatation, with the risk of ischaemia and perforation. An incompetent ileocaecal valve allows colonic decompression, with passage of air into the small bowel. Onset of symptoms may then be more gradual.

AXR

On supine AXR, look for:

• Dilated gas-filled colon proximal to the site of obstruction (Fig. 6.2)
• Paucity of gas in collapsed colon distal to the obstruction
• Haustral pattern to differentiate from small bowel

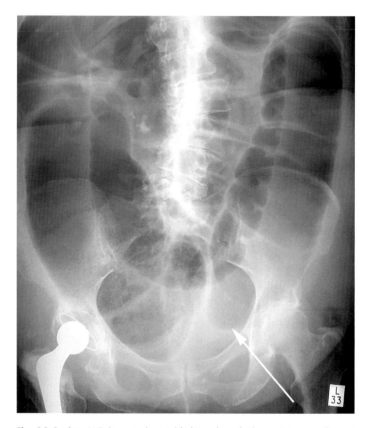

Fig. 6.2 Supine AXR in a patient with large bowel obstruction secondary to sigmoid carcinoma. There is gaseous distension of the large bowel down to the left pelvis at level of obstruction (arrow).

- Small bowel dilatation also if ileocaecal valve incompetent
- Evidence of perforation.

If large bowel obstruction is diagnosed, rectal and sigmoidoscopic examination should be performed to exclude a low obstructing lesion. If negative, the patient should be considered for contrast enema examination of the large bowel.

CXR

On erect CXR, look for evidence of free intraperitoneal air, lung metastases and other pathology.

Contrast enema

Although barium is the ideal agent, it can cause problems. It is contraindicated in patients at risk of perforation and can cause impaction if no obstruction is present, as well as interfering with future colonoscopy and CT (see Chapter 2). Iodinated contrast (water-soluble) is often used and will exclude gross obstruction (Fig. 6.3).

CT

This can be useful in assessing bowel and adjacent structures, particularly if patients are elderly or frail and cannot tolerate a contrast enema.

Pseudo-obstruction

Marked dilatation of the large bowel may occur in elderly, bedridden patients or those with neurological or psychiatric disorders. Gaseous distension often involves the rectum also, and faecal loading may be present. Sigmoidoscopy and contrast enema are often needed to exclude a mechanical obstruction in patients who do not settle with conservative treatment.

Diverticular disease of the colon

This is the most common colonic disease in the West, with diverticula present in up to 50% of people of 50 years of age, with the sigmoid colon most frequently involved. Diverticula are out-pouchings of colonic mucosa and submucosa that penetrate between circular muscle fibres. Circular muscle hypertrophy and muscular spasm are common. Diverticular disease is generally diagnosed during barium enema examination, often as an incidental finding (Fig. 6.4). Complications of diverticular disease include diverticulitis, fistula formation and haemorrhage.

Diverticulitis

Diverticulitis is the most common complication of diverticular disease, occurring in up to 25% of patients. It occurs secondary to mucosal abrasion by faecal matter within a diverticulum, causing local perforation, inflammation and abscess formation. Patients present with left iliac fossa pain, fever and often an inflammatory mass.

AXR

AXR may demonstrate air within an abscess or secondary ileus. Chronic inflammation and stricturing with large bowel obstruction is unusual.

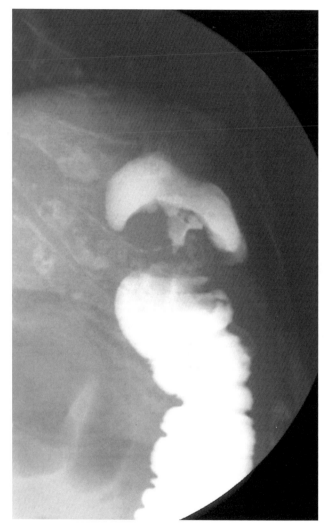

Fig. 6.3 Water-soluble contrast enema film from splenic flexure region shows an obstructing carcinoma. Note 'apple core' appearance of stricture with shouldering.

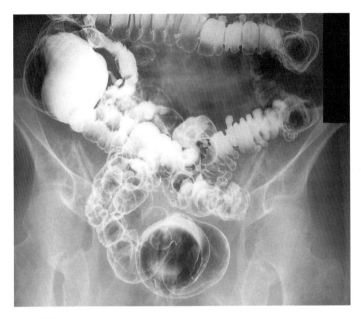

Fig. 6.4 Film from double-contrast barium enema series showing florid sigmoid diverticular disease. Note diverticula and circular muscle hypertrophy. The sigmoid colon is tortuous and is an area of weakness for barium enema—mucosal lesions can easily be overlooked. Another problem here is the presence of significant small bowel reflux of barium, which partially obscures the sigmoid region.

Barium enema

This is excellent at demonstrating diverticular colonic muscular hypertrophy and spasm, and local contrast extravasation into walled-off pericolic abscess. Patients often do not tolerate barium enema during an acute episode, and enema does not delineate pericolic inflammation.

US

US is often requested as a first-line investigation for patients with left iliac fossa pain and may demonstrate bowel-wall thickening, a mass or fluid collection in diverticulitis. However, US is often non-diagnostic.

CT

Patients often proceed to CT, which accurately delineates diverticula, bowel-wall thickening, pericolic inflammatory change and abscess formation (Fig. 6.5), and will guide aspiration or drainage of abscess.

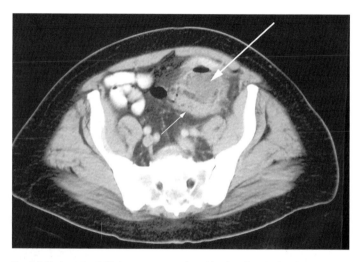

Fig. 6.5 Post-contrast CT demonstrates a sigmoid colon diverticular abscess. There is an irregular mass containing fluid and air (long arrow). Thick-walled sigmoid colon abuts the abscess (short arrow).

Note:
It is important to remember that perforated carcinoma can mimic diverticulitis, and once the acute episode has settled, patients should undergo endoscopic examination.

Fistula formation

A fistula is a communication between two surfaces lined by epithelium. A colovesical fistula is the commonest type of indiverticular disease and is secondary to recurrent inflammation — these patients present with pneumaturia. Air in the bladder may be apparent on AXR. The fistula can be demarcated during barium enema. CT is very sensitive at detecting air in the bladder, with associated changes in the sigmoid colon. Coloenteric (Fig. 6.6), colovaginal and colocutaneous fistulae may also occur.

Remember that fistula formation also occurs with malignancy and this should be excluded.

Haemorrhage

This is not related to diverticulitis. It occurs in 30–50% of patients with diverticular disease and may be life-threatening. Haemorrhage is usually self-limiting, but re-bleeding is common.

Barium enema or colonoscopy is indicated if bleeding is to be investigated as an outpatient. Catastrophic haemorrhage may require angiography to iden-

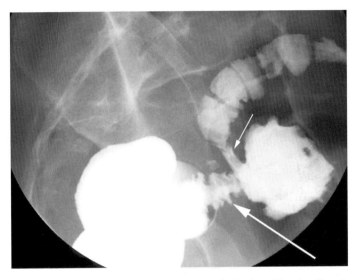

Fig. 6.6 Film from a single-contrast barium enema in the sigmoid region. There is irregular narrowing in the mid-sigmoid region (long arrow) with adjacent diverticular disease. Contrast passes via a fistula (short arrow) to communicate with small bowel. This was secondary to diverticular disease, but exclusion of malignancy is essential.

tify the site and to allow potential embolization of the bleeding vessel.

Colorectal carcinoma

Colorectal carcinoma is the second most common cause of cancer death. Risk factors include family history, adenomatous polyposis syndromes, chronic ulcerative colitis and Crohn's disease. The vast majority of colorectal carcinomas begin as benign adenomas, which grow over time and undergo malignant transformation. Adenomas of >1 cm are at risk and >2 cm malignancy is likely

(50%). Fifty per cent of carcinomas are in the rectum or sigmoid and in range of the flexible sigmoidoscope.

Patients with a colorectal carcinoma are at risk of synchronous (carcinoma elsewhere in large bowel) and metachronous (colonic carcinoma at a later date) lesions and it is important to evaluate the entire colon at the time of diagnosis.

Polyp detection

Clearly, polyp detection and removal prior to malignant change is essential for prevention of colorectal carcinoma, although large-scale population screening

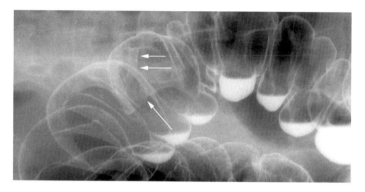

Fig. 6.7 Decubitus spot film of the hepatic flexure from a double-contrast barium enema series demonstrates a pedunculated polyp on a stalk (arrows). Note gravitational pooling of barium.

is still under investigation. Several imaging modalities are available; all have strengths and weaknesses. Colonoscopy is often preferred.

Barium enema

Double-contrast barium enema is highly accurate and comparable to colonoscopy in the identification of polyps >1 cm. This accuracy falls off <1 cm in size. Completion rate to the caecum is better with barium enema. Diagnostic accuracy is impaired:
• With poor bowel preparation
• If patients cannot retain air or barium
• With tortuosity of the bowel, especially in the sigmoid
• With extensive associated diverticular disease
• The lower rectum is often not well seen, particularly if a balloon catheter is used.

Adenomatous polyps may be:
• *Pedunculated* (on a stalk): where risk of malignancy is low (Fig. 6.7)
• *Sessile* (flat): villous change and malignancy is more likely (Fig. 6.8).

Colonoscopy

Endoscopic assessment of the colon allows identification and also removal of polyps. This modality is theoretically the ideal, but does have the complications of sedation and perforation, and technical failure is common, for similar reasons, to barium enema.

CT colonography

This three-dimensional virtual-reality CT technique, following air insufflation of the colon, has shown initial promising results.

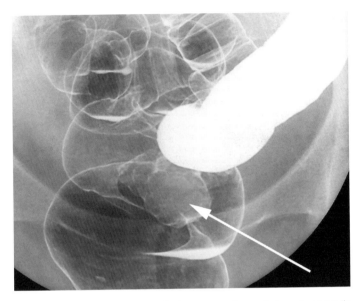

Fig. 6.8 Film from double-contrast barium enema demonstrates a large sessile polyp in the upper rectum (arrow). The surface of the polyp is irregular and, when combined with the size, malignancy is likely.

Adenocarcinoma

This may be diagnosed by the three modalities outlined above — again, colonoscopy offers the opportunity for histological examination.

Barium enema

Look for:
- Fungating, polypoidal lesion
- Annular, ulcerating — 'apple core' with shouldering (Fig. 6.9)
- Scirrhous lesion (uncommon).

CT

CT is useful for identifying primary tumour and is the most reliable method for staging:
- Luminal mass and bowel wall thickening (Fig. 6.10)
- Stranding and nodularity of adjacent fat — may indicate local invasion
- Invasion of local structures
- Presence of mesenteric disease, ascites, significant adenopathy
- Liver and lung metastases.

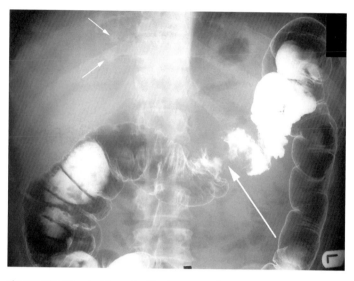

Fig. 6.9 Film from double-contrast barium enema in a patient with a large transverse colon carcinoma (large arrow). There is irregular stricturing of the bowel with shouldering apparent. Note lung metastases at lung bases (small arrows).

US

Transabdominal US can identify bowel-related masses and will assess the liver parenchyma for metastases.

Transrectal US and MRI accurately delineate the layers of the rectal wall and are useful for local staging of disease. Bulky and locally invasive rectal carcinomas will receive local radiotherapy prior to surgery.

Local complications of colorectal carcinoma

• *Obstruction:* this is common (see earlier). In patients unfit for immediate

surgery, radiological insertion of an expanding metallic stent over a guidewire can relieve obstruction, giving palliation. Surgery can be considered when the patient's condition has improved.
• *Fistula formation* (see earlier)
• *Perforation:* patients may go straight to theatre for surgery.

Follow-up of treated colorectal cancer

Residual large bowel post-resection is followed-up regularly, either endoscopically or by barium enema.

CT is the modality currently of choice for identifying extraluminal local recur-

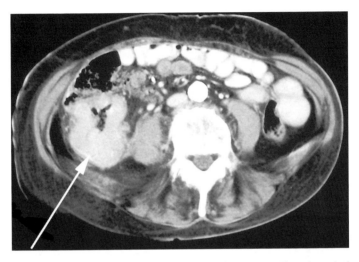

Fig. 6.10 Post-contrast CT in a patient with caecal carcinoma. There is marked thickening of the caecal wall (arrows).

rence or metastatic disease and is also used to monitor patients with known metastatic disease undergoing treatment.

Hepatic metastases may be considered for ablation or resection (see Chapter 7).

Abdominal sepsis

Sepsis in the abdomen is a very important cause of patient mortality, morbidity and increased length of hospital stay. Cases are often complex and great benefit may be obtained through direct discussion with a radiologist.

This section concentrates on intraperitoneal, subphrenic, psoas and pelvic abscess formation. Diverticular, pancreatic and hepatic abscesses are covered elsewhere.

Intraperitoneal abscess

Usually results from secondary infection of collections of blood, bile or ascites and may arise in patients who have undergone bowel or hepatobiliary surgery. If patients have pyrexia or a raised white cell count only, with no significant abdominal symptoms, make sure there is no evidence of chest, urinary or skin sepsis (e.g. infected cannula) prior to further investigations.

AXR

AXR may show an ileus or mottled

gas densities within an intraperitoneal abscess and is worth arranging if there are abdominal symptoms.

US

US is the next investigation of choice for the identification of abdominal and pelvic fluid collections. Bandaging, suturing, pain, obesity and gas often degrade US; CT would then be recommended.

Percutaneous drainage under US or CT guidance can be performed in post-operative abscess formation.

Subphrenic abscess

This usually follows bowel surgery or appendicectomy.

AXR

AXR may show mottled gas densities in abscess but air–fluid level and sympathetic pleural effusion is best appreciated on erect CXR (Fig. 6.11).

US and CT

US or CT will confirm diagnosis if necessary.

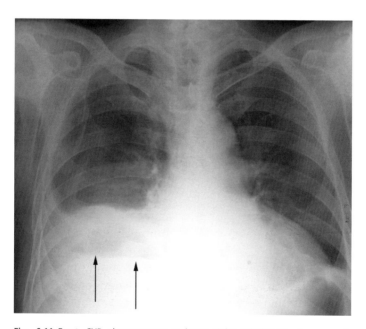

Fig. 6.11 Erect CXR demonstrates a large right subphrenic abscess post-cholecystectomy. Note air–fluid level (arrows) and right basal pleural effusion.

Psoas abscess

Psoas abscess often relates to adjacent vertebral, bowel or renal sepsis. Look for evidence clinically of psoas irritation and painful hip flexion.

AXR

AXR may show psoas enlargement and abnormal gas densities. Look carefully for renal tract calcification and vertebral body abnormality (tuberculous or metastatic bony involvement).

US and CT

US is often limited in evaluation of the retroperitoneum and CT is the ideal modality for psoas assessment and abscess drainage (Fig. 6.12).

Colitis

The three most common forms of colitis are dealt with here: ulcerative, Crohn's and ischaemic.

Ulcerative colitis

This is a common inflammatory disease of the colon and rectum of uncertain aetiology, which initially involves the bowel mucosa but extends to involve deeper layers. The disease usually commences in the rectum and extends proximally, with the diagnosis made on sigmoidoscopic biopsy. The terminal ileum may be involved ('backwash ileitis').

Ulcerative colitis runs a variable clinical course—usually with periods of

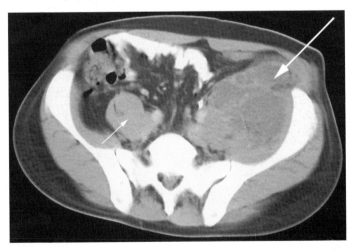

Fig. 6.12 CT of left psoas abscess secondary to renal calculus disease. A large septated fluid collection involves the left psoas and iliacus muscles (long arrow). Note normal right psoas muscle (short arrow).

relapse and remission, although an acute and fulminant illness may occur. Extra-colonic manifestations are recognised (e.g. arthritis, iritis, rash) in 10%.

AXR

Look for:
• Extent of faecal residue—where it is absent this is suggestive of colitic involvement
• Bowel wall thickening
• Colon diameter (>6 cm in traverse colon suspicious of toxic megacolon). Colon narrows in chronic disease
• Loss of haustration or mural thickening
• Evidence of perforation.

Barium enema

This is a useful investigation in ulcerative colitis. It is used to assess disease extent, to differentiate ulcerative colitis from other forms of colitis and to detect disease complications (e.g. malignancy).

Barium enema features of ulcerative colitis

Acute changes
Granular mucosa pattern
'Collar-stud' ulcers (shallow ulceration underlying mucosa)
Haustral thickening ('thumb-printing')
Inflammatory polyps

Chronic changes (Fig. 6.13)
Haustral loss
Colon shortening
Luminal narrowing ('lead-pipe' colon)

Postinflammatory polyps
Terminal ileitis

Complications of ulcerative colitis

• *Toxic megacolon:* an acute fulminant illness with colonic dilatation (>6 cm) and high risk of perforation. It carries a high mortality. Toxic megacolon can be diagnosed on AXR (Fig. 6.14). Contrast enema should not be performed because of the risk of perforation.
• *Colonic adenocarcinoma:* annual incidence of 10% after first decade of the disease. Carcinomas are often multiple and flat, and scirrhous in nature (Fig. 6.13). Patients with ulcerative colitis should undergo regular colonoscopic screening with random biopsies to detect dysplasia.

Crohn's colitis (see Chapter 5)

This is a granulomatous colitis particularly involving the right colon, with sparing of rectum and sigmoid colon. However, perianal disease (abscess, fistula, ulceration) is strongly suggestive of Crohn's.

AXR

Look for:
• Extent of faecal residue, bowel-wall thickening, haustral loss or thickening (Fig. 6.15)
• Also look for gallstones, sacroiliitis and avascular necrosis (femoral heads), which are associated with Crohn's (and ulcerative colitis).

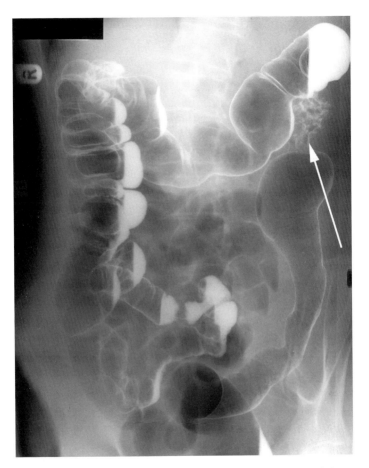

Fig. 6.13 Films from double-contrast barium enema in a patient with long-standing ulcerative colitis involving the colon around to the hepatic flexure. Note granular mucosa with colon lumen narrowed and haustral pattern absent. A complicating carcinoma is seen at the splenic flexure (arrow). Note normal haustral pattern in the right colon.

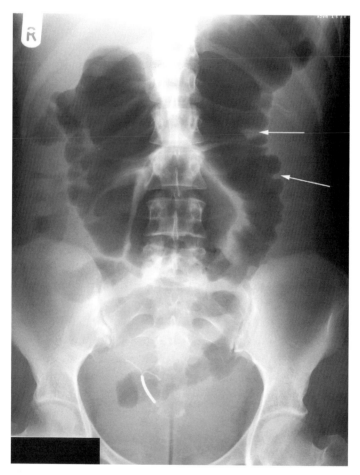

Fig. 6.14 AXR in a patient with ulcerative pancolitis and toxic dilatation of the transverse colon. Note absence of faecal residue and thickening of haustra (arrows). There is a pelvic intrauterine contraceptive device (IUCD).

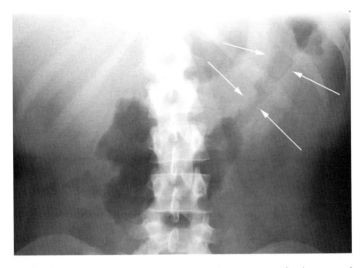

Fig. 6.15 AXR in a patient with Crohn's colitis. The transverse colon is narrowed and thumb-printing (mucosal oedema) is present (arrows).

Barium enema features of Crohn's colitis

Early
Nodular lymphoid hyperplasia
Aphthous ulcers
'Cobblestoning' resulting from longi-
   tudinal and transverse ulcers sepa-
   rated by oedema — ulcers are deep
Thickened haustra
Inflammatory pseudopolyps
Discontinuous involvement ('skip
   lesions')

Late
Loss of haustration
Strictures ('string' sign)
Fistulae
Pseudodiverticula

Complications of Crohn's colitis

• *Fistula:* enterocolic, enterocutaneous,
perianal
• *Toxic megacolon:* less common than
ulcerative colitis
• *Adenocarcinoma:* ileum and colon
• *Abscess formation.*

Ischaemic colitis

Patients present with acute abdominal
pain and rectal bleeding, and ischaemic
colitis tends to involve the splenic flexure
and descending colon at the 'watershed'
area of blood supply between superior
and inferior mesenteric arteries. It is
more common in the elderly with a
history of cardiovascular disease.

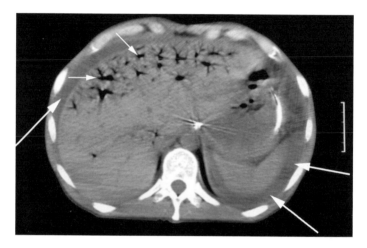

Fig. 6.16 Post-contrast CT in a severely ill patient with ischaemic colitis. Air is identified peripherally distributed within portal veins in the liver (small arrows). Ascites is present (large arrows).

AXR

AXR may show segmental mucosal oedema with thumb-printing. Diagnosis can be confirmed with barium enema.

CT

CT demonstrates segmental mural thickening, and also intramural and portal venous gas in severely ill patients (Fig. 6.16).

Caecal volvulus

Caecal volvulus accounts for 3% of colonic obstructions and is associated with malrotation of the right colon and a long mesentery allowing the caecum to rotate so it lies in the mid-abdomen or, more commonly, the left upper quadrant.

AXR

AXR reveals a dilated gas-filled caecum in the left upper quadrant (Fig. 6.17). The medially placed ileocaecal valve may cause an indentation, giving a kidney or 'coffee-bean' appearance.

If the ileocaecal valve is incompetent, there will be coexisting small bowel dilatation. The normal caecal gas pattern is absent in the right iliac fossa.

A contrast enema is helpful if AXR is atypical, with the tapered end of the obstructed contrast column pointing toward the torsion.

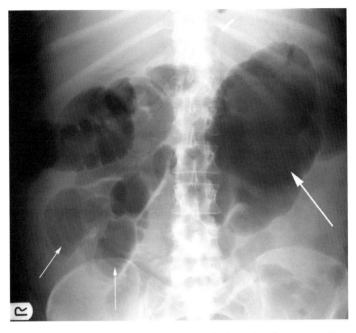

Fig. 6.17 Supine AXR in a patient with caecal volvulus and an incompetent ileocaecal valve. Note distended air-filled caecum in left upper quadrant (large arrow) and dilated small bowel loops (small arrows).

Sigmoid volvulus

This accounts for 1–2% of colonic obstructions and tends to occur in elderly or psychiatric patients with large redundant sigmoid colons.

Patients present with abdominal pain and distension.

AXR

On supine AXR, look for:
• Markedly dilated loop of sigmoid colon extending into the upper abdomen, converging to the left iliac fossa (Fig. 6.18)
• Often dilated large bowel proximally
• Absence of gas in the rectum.

A contrast enema may be required in some patients where radiographical findings are equivocal. This demonstrates a tapered narrowing of the contrast column at level of volvulus.

Once the diagnosis has been made, a flatus tube can be passed to decompress the sigmoid colon to allow patient stabilization prior to sigmoid colectomy.

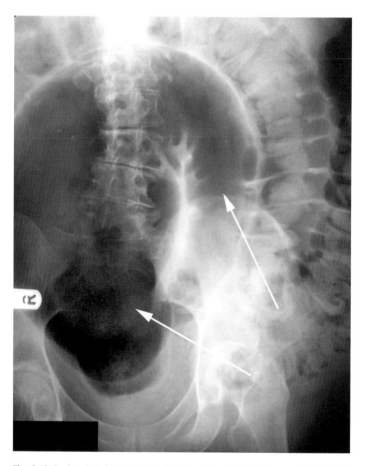

Fig. 6.18 Supine AXR in a patient with sigmoid volvulus. Note markedly dilated sigmoid colon (arrows) with 'inverted-U' configuration, converging to the left iliac fossa. Calcified gallstones are seen in the right upper quadrant.

Further reading

Gore RM, Levine MS, eds. *Textbook of Gastrointestinal Radiology*, 2nd edn. Philadelphia: Saunders, 2000.

Levine MS, Rubesin SE, Laufer I, eds. *Double Contrast Gastrointestinal Radiology*, 3rd edn. Philadelphia: Saunders, 2000.

Miller FH, ed. *The Radiological Clinics of North America: Radiology of the Pancreas, Gall bladder and Biliary Tract*, Vol. 40. 2002.

Chapter 7: **Hepatobiliary and pancreatic imaging**

This chapter covers:

Common conditions
- Gallstones and their complications
- Hepatic metastases
- Hepatic abscess
- Cirrhosis
- Acute and chronic pancreatitis
- Carcinoma of the pancreas
- Bile duct stricture
- Abdominal trauma

Common presentations in which imaging can help
- Acute abdominal pain: gallstones, cholecystitis, pancreatitis
- Chronic abdominal pain: gallstones, hepatomegaly (cirrhosis, metastases, hepatitis)
- Jaundice: obstructive or hepatic
- Non-specific symptoms also occur in many conditions (e.g. nausea, vomiting, weight loss, malaise)

Imaging strategy

Imaging will depend on the initial working differential diagnosis, taking into account results of blood tests, patient age and previous medical history.

The general principles of imaging apply. Investigations should be tailored to each patient and the use of ionizing radiation kept to a minimum. The use of relatively non-invasive investigations, US and MRI, should be encouraged.

Discussion of individual cases with a radiologist is often extremely helpful in this area and will allow prioritization and ease of access.

When admitted acutely with upper abdominal pain and vomiting, most patients will have a supine AXR and erect CXR performed, as perforated viscus is often important in the differential diagnosis.

AXR

AXR gives often limited diagnostic information relating to the liver, biliary tree and pancreas. Look for hepatomegaly, abnormal patterns of calcification, bowel gas pattern, abnormal distribution of air (e.g. in gall bladder wall or biliary tree). If you are unsure, ask a senior colleague.

US

Following initial clinical assessment and plain radiography, US is frequently requested.

US as a modality has significant advantages:
- It is readily available
- It is safe, with no ionizing radiation
- It is accurate in assessing the biliary tree, the gall bladder for mass or stones and the hepatic parenchyma.

However, US does have some drawbacks:
- It is operator dependent.
- It is patient dependent. Patient

obesity or large amounts of bowel gas often significantly degrade the image. The pancreas in particular is often poorly seen, unless an endoscopic technique is used.

US is a good screening tool, however, and a *normal*, good quality examination may obviate the need for further imaging.

CT

CT is the investigation of choice for several conditions, particularly if initial US is equivocal. Focal liver lesions and the pancreas are well-demonstrated with CT, as is the retroperitoneum and mesentery.

CT involves significant amounts of ionizing radiation and usually also requires administration of oral and intravenous iodinated contrast. Patient cooperation with breath-holding is important.

CT and US can be used to guide biopsy and drainage procedures (see Table 7).

MR

The advent of high-quality MR units and magnetic resonance cholangiopancreatography (MRCP) has had a significant impact on hepatobiliary imaging. MRCP has largely replaced diagnostic endoscopic retrograde cholangiopancreatography (ERCP) in many centres. MR is used often as problem-solving tool following initial US and CT.

MR does not involve ionizing radiation or iodinated contrast and can be used instead of CT in certain patients (e.g. young, iodine allergy). MR does have some contraindications (see Chapter 2), and claustrophobia may be a problem.

NM

NM is not generally used as a first-line investigation for the liver, biliary tree or pancreas, and will not be covered in detail in this chapter.

Diseases of the gall bladder

Gallstones are common and most frequently occur in overweight middle-aged females. Stones are usually cholesterol-based, although pigment stones do occur. This section concentrates on the complications of gallstone disease and how imaging may assist in diagnosis and management.

Acute cholecystitis

Patients most commonly present with acute right upper quadrant pain on a background of more chronic biliary symptoms. The vast majority of cases are secondary to calculus impaction in the cystic duct, with gall bladder outflow obstruction and secondary bacterial infection (10% of cases are acalculous).

Imaging is important to:
• Confirm the diagnosis and exclude other causes of right upper quadrant pain
• Evaluate potential complications (see below).

AXR

AXR can provide useful diagnostic information and is generally performed (supine) on admission. About 10% of calculi are radio-opaque on radiographs because of calcium content, and some complications of cholecystitis (e.g.

air–calcium in gall bladder wall or ileus) may be apparent.

US

This represents the imaging modality of choice for the evaluation of suspected gallstones and cholecystitis, with reported accuracies of >95%. Gallstones are seen as hyperechoic foci with distal acoustic shadowing. Sonographic changes of acute cholecystitis include (Fig. 7.1):
• Positive Murphy's sign during scanning
• Gallstones in the gall bladder
• Gall bladder wall thickening, with or without free fluid.

The accuracy of US is reduced in the obese, in patients with extreme tenderness preventing examination and in the presence of large amounts of bowel gas.

CT

CT is not generally used in the initial assessment of acute cholecystitis but may be useful if complications (e.g. gall bladder perforation with or without abscess) are suspected. CT is less accurate than US in the detection of calculi.

NM

Cholescintigraphy is accurate in the assessment of acute cholecystitis, but its

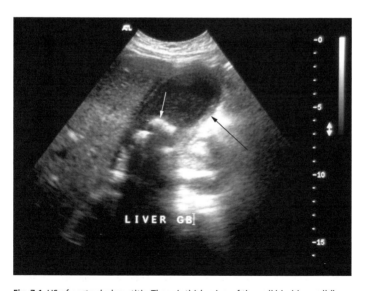

Fig. 7.1 US of acute cholecystitis. There is thickening of the gall bladder wall (long black arrow) and stones are seen in the gall bladder (short white arrow) with acoustic shadowing in association.

use is generally limited to cases with negative sonography.

Complications of acute cholecystitis

Gall bladder empyema and perforation

Cystic duct obstruction secondary to calculus or oedema may cause gall bladder distension (mucocele) and infection may supervene to produce an empyema.

Ultrasound features of empyema include gall bladder calculi or sludge, and pronounced mural thickening. These patients are at high risk of perforation.

Ultrasound- or CT-guided drainage of gall bladder empyema should be considered in patients unfit for immediate surgery.

Emphysematous cholecystitis (rare)

This is caused by calculus or oedematous obstruction of the cystic duct with secondary ischaemia of the gall bladder wall and infection with gas-forming organisms (e.g. *Clostridium perfringens*). Diabetics are predisposed and mortality is high.

On AXR, look for air in the gall bladder wall and air–fluid level in the gall bladder. With US, look for calculi and air in the gall bladder wall.

Chronic cholecystitis

This is caused by recurrent episodes of acute inflammation secondary to calculi and intermittent cystic duct obstruction. It may be difficult to differentiate clinically the contraction of a chronically inflamed gall bladder from acute inflammation.

AXR

Look for calcified gallstones, calcified gall bladder wall (Fig. 7.2) and radio-opaque bile resulting from calcium carbonate ('limy bile').

US

Look for calculi and contracted thick-walled gall bladder.

Complications of chronic cholelithiasis

Porcelain gall bladder

This is rare, resulting from chronic inflammation of the gall bladder wall with calcification. It is associated with gallstones and malignancy.
• *AXR:* calcification in gall bladder wall (Fig. 7.2)
• *US/CT:* calcification and carcinoma as luminal mass.

Gallstone ileus

This occurs in chronic cholecystitis with erosion of calculus into the gastrointestinal tract. Stone impaction may occur, with obstruction at areas of luminal narrowing (e.g. ileocaecal valve).
• *AXR:* look for triad of air in biliary tree, dilated small bowel loops and gallstone within bowel loop (Fig. 7.3). The calculus is often not seen if radiolucent and surrounded by fluid. Biliary tree air does not extend to the liver edge and tends to have a central/portal distribution.

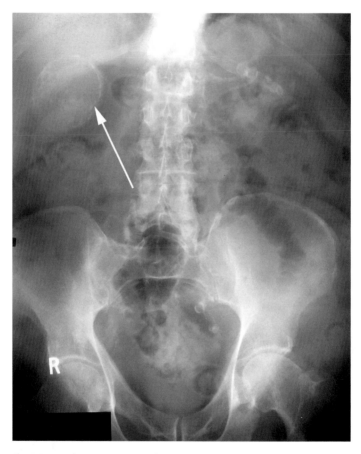

Fig. 7.2 AXR demonstrating curvilinear calcification of the gall bladder wall in porcelain gall bladder (arrow).

Gall bladder carcinoma

This has strong association with gall-stones and patients present with symptoms of right upper quadrant pain, weight loss and jaundice.

• *US:* useful initially and may show a gall bladder mass, bile duct dilatation and liver metastases. However, access may be limited (see above).
• *CT/MR:* used for further assessment and accurate in the detection of local

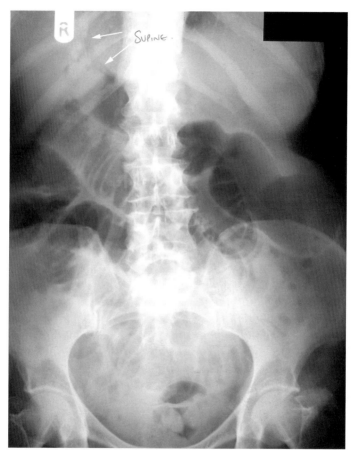

Fig. 7.3 AXR of gallstone ileus. There are dilated loops of small bowel with air in the biliary tree (arrows). A calcified gallstone is not identified but a stone was found impacted at the ileocaecal valve at laparotomy.

liver invasion and extrahepatic nodal disease in addition, rendering lesions inoperable.

Choledocholithiasis

Ninety-five per cent of patients with common duct calculi have gallstones in the gall bladder and 15% of patients with gallstones also have stones in the common duct.

Presenting features of choledocholithiasis include pain, sepsis, pancreatitis or jaundice.

AXR

AXR may visualize stones (10% are radio-opaque).

US

This is the most useful initial imaging modality, but degradation due to bowel gas is important and up to one-third of distal duct stones are missed. US is accurate in the assessment of intrahepatic and common duct dilatation and guides the need for further imaging.

MRCP

This uses a fast T2-weighted sequence, where bile is high signal and stones are seen as filling defects (Fig. 7.4). It is highly accurate for the demonstration of duct stones and has replaced diagnostic ERCP in many centres.

ERCP

Is accurate in the detection of common duct stones and allows therapeutic intervention (e.g. stent placement, sphincterotomy) but is invasive. Complications include pancreatitis, cholangitis or perforation and haemorrhage post-sphincterotomy.

CT

CT is less accurate in the detection of common duct stones, and a combination of US and MRCP is more frequently used.

Cholangiography

The ducts can be visualized and stones detected intra-operatively by direct iodinated contrast injection into the duct (on-table cholangiogram), or postoperatively if a T-tube is in place (T-tube cholangiogram; Fig. 7.5).

Hepatic metastases

The liver is the most common metastatic site after regional lymph nodes. Colon, stomach, pancreas, breast and lung are the leading primary sites. The most common clinical presentations are hepatomegaly, jaundice and ascites. Liver function tests are often normal and accurate imaging is essential in diagnosis, treatment and follow-up.

The characteristics of metastases may need to be differentiated from other diseases of the liver and a careful imaging strategy is needed, usually formulated following discussion with a radiologist.

AXR

Look for hepatomegaly, ascites and punctate amorphous calcifications,

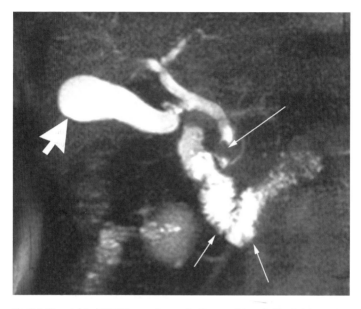

Fig. 7.4 T2-weighted MRCP image demonstrating a gallstone in the distal common bile duct, seen as a low signal filling defect (long arrow). Note normal gall bladder (arrowhead) and duodenal loop (small arrows).

which may occur in colloid carcinoma metastases (stomach, colon). Do remember to request a CXR also in suspected metastatic disease.

US

This is the initial investigation of choice and is accurate in identifying focal liver lesions. Metastases have varying sonographical appearances (Fig. 7.6).

CT

CT is frequently used for further evalua-

tion of focal lesions and if US is non-diagnostic (Fig. 7.7). US and CT can both be used to guide percutaneous biopsy of a lesion to obtain histological confirmation of the diagnosis (Table 7.1). Hepatocellular carcinoma and lymphoma may both appear similar to metastasis and treatment options differ—if clinically appropriate, histological examination should always be performed.

Certain liver metastases may be treated with image-guided ablation techniques or surgical resection. If these are contemplated then further imaging—either CT angiography and portography

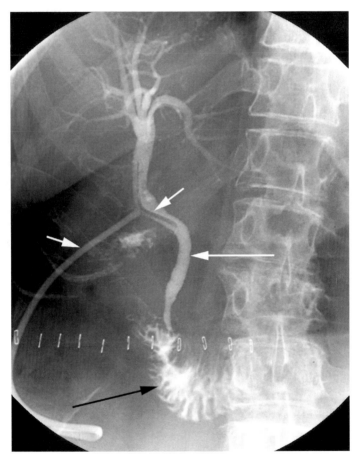

Fig. 7.5 Normal T-tube cholangiogram study. Iodinated contrast is injected down the T-tube (short white arrows) and opacifies the duct system and ampulla passing into the duodenum (black arrow). The common bile duct is indicated by a long white arrow.

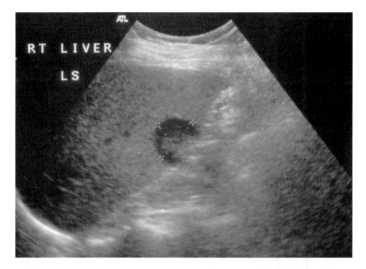

Fig. 7.6 US of the liver in a patient with known breast cancer. A focal hypoechoic lesion (callipers) is present in the right lobe of the liver, consistent with metastasis.

Table 7.1 Liver biopsy: CT- or US-guided.

Can be used to biopsy
Focal lesions
Diffusely abnormal liver, but no focal lesion
Macroscopically normal liver, but biochemical abnormality

Contraindications
Patient unable to give informed consent or unable to cooperate
Presence of ascites (can drain prior to procedure)
Bleeding diathesis (prolonged prothrombin or activated partial thromboplastin time, platelet count <100 000/mL). Discuss with haematology and radiology departments. It may still be possible to biopsy with covering transfusion with fresh frozen plasma or platelets. Blind biopsy can be performed via transjugular route if severe clotting derangement

Patient preparation
Nil by mouth
Intravenous access
Consent
Check full blood count, coagulation profile, group and save

Complications
Minor ache or shoulder discomfort is common post-procedure
Haemorrhage (rarely significant), or bile leak (rare)
Pneumothorax

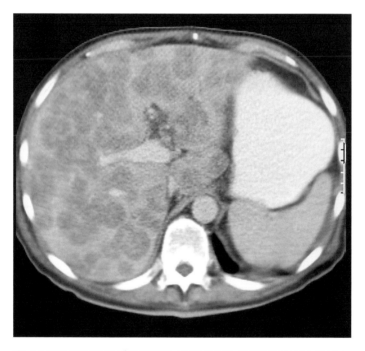

Fig. 7.7 Post-contrast CT of the liver in a patient with colonic carcinoma. The liver contains multiple hypodense metastases.

(CTAP), or MR would be performed to exclude other lesions. CTAP involves direct iodinated contrast injection via a catheter placed into the hepatic, splenic or superior mesenteric artery and then imaging the liver.

Hepatic abscess

Pyogenic liver abscess can arise from five main routes:

1 Biliary (obstructed duct system, stones) — the most common cause
2 Portal venous (bowel inflammation)
3 Hepatic arterial (septicaemia)
4 Direct extension from adjacent organ
5 Traumatic penetrating injury.

Escherichia coli and streptococci are the main causative organisms in adults. Abscesses are usually multiple and presenting features may be vague. Tender hepatomegaly and deranged liver function tests are common.

CXR

This is often abnormal. Look for elevation of right hemidiaphragm, right basal atelectasis or pleural effusion.

AXR

Look for gas or air–fluid level overlying the liver.

US

US is highly sensitive and demonstrates hypoechoic lesions down to 1–1.5 cm and may identify foci of air within abscesses. However, US is not specific, and differential diagnosis includes necrotic tumours, haematoma, complex cyst or biloma.

CT

This is the most accurate modality. Abscesses appear rounded and hypodense, often with an enhancing rim. Air within abscesses may be seen and multiple small abscesses may cluster into a larger lesion (Fig. 7.8).

Interventional treatment

For small unilocular suspected abscesses, aspiration under CT or US guidance may suffice together with antibiotic therapy. Discuss with the radiologist. For larger or complex lesions, formal guided drainage is required (Fig. 7.9), and large drains (up to 16 French) may be needed if pus is thick. Surgery may be needed if catheter drainage fails or if there is associated fistula formation (biliary or colonic).

It is important to investigate for an underlying cause of the abscess. Do not forget to send samples to microbiology. It is often helpful to discuss the case with a microbiologist. Patient preparation and complications for abscess drainage are similar to those for liver biopsy in Table 7.1.

Cirrhosis

Alcohol is the most common cause of liver cirrhosis, with viral hepatitis and biliary cirrhosis the other more common causes. Patients may present with vague upper abdominal symptoms, hepatomegaly or abnormal liver function tests, or with complications of the disease (e.g. liver failure, portal hypertension, ascites, hepatocellular carcinoma).

US

This is most commonly used for initial assessment. Many sonographical findings are non-specific but certain features are suggestive:
- Small liver with nodular surface
- Coarse texture
- Evidence of portal hypertension (ascites, splenomegaly, varices)
- Can guide ascitic tap or drainage.

CT

CT is useful for further evaluation (Fig. 7.10) and particularly for:
- Poorly visualized liver or very coarse liver texture on US
- Focal lesion(s) on US
- Clinical or biochemical suspicion of hepatocellular carcinoma.

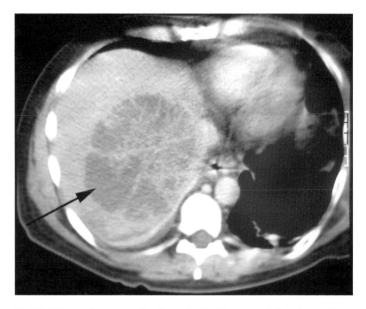

Fig. 7.8 CT image through the liver in a patient with a pyogenic liver abscess. There is a large hypodense lesion (arrow) comprising multiple small abscesses clustered together.

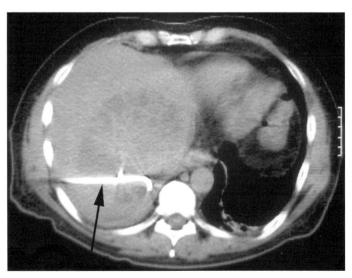

Fig. 7.9 CT image of the abscess in the same patient as Fig. 7.8, following percutaneous insertion of a pigtail drainage catheter (arrow).

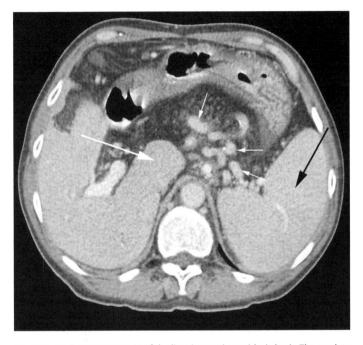

Fig. 7.10 Axial post-contrast CT of the liver in a patient with cirrhosis. The caudate lobe is enlarged (large white arrow). The liver surface is irregular, the spleen is enlarged (black arrow) and varices are present (small white arrows).

Pancreatitis

Acute pancreatitis

Alcohol and gallstone disease are the most common aetiologies. Clinical findings are often non-specific, but include varying degrees of abdominal pain, nausea and vomiting. Serum amylase measurement may be helpful — although amylase can be elevated in other conditions including perforated duodenal ulcer and may be normal in severe necrotizing pancreatitis.

What is the role of imaging?
• To exclude other pathologies as cause of symptoms
• To confirm diagnosis of acute pancreatitis
• To evaluate the degree of pancreatic injury and presence of complications (e.g. abscess).

AXR

Look for duodenal ileus (sentinel loop is an overlying dilated gas-filled small bowel loop) or, rarely, gas bubbles in a pancreatic abscess.

CXR

Look for elevated hemidiaphragm, atelectasis or pleural effusion.

US

US is useful in patients with mild disease and those with a suspected gallstone aetiology.

US may demonstrate hypoechoic swelling of the gland and associated fluid collections. However, US is limited, often by bowel gas, and CT is required for more severe disease.

CT

This is the most useful test in clinically severe acute pancreatitis. It:
• Assesses the gland (Fig. 7.11) and, by lack of contrast enhancement, can identify areas of necrosis
• Visualizes the retroperitoneum, mesentery and omentum
• Accurately delineates associated fluid collections, pseudocyst and abscess for-

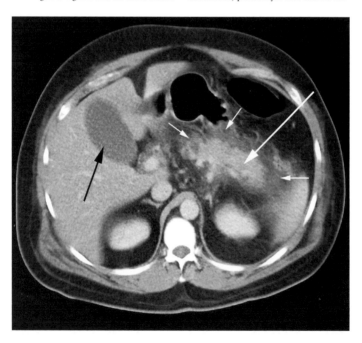

Fig. 7.11 Post-contrast CT through the pancreatic body and tail in a patient with acute pancreatitis. The pancreas is enlarged and poorly defined (large white arrow), but enhances homogeneously. Note associated inflammatory changes in the adjacent mesenteric fat (small white arrows) and normal gall bladder (black arrow).

mation (Fig. 7.12) and can be used to guide therapeutic aspiration or drainage.

Chronic pancreatitis

Alcohol is the major risk factor, and pain radiating to the back with weight loss are the most common symptoms. Diabetes and malabsorption develop in some patients.

AXR

Small irregular pancreatic calcifications occur in up to 50% of patients and are pathognomic (Fig. 7.13).

US

US can provide useful information concerning gland morphology, calcification and duct dilatation but is often limited because of technical factors. It may demonstrate a pseudocyst.

CT

CT accurately delineates the gland and areas of atrophy, or focal enlargement. Focal enlargement can be difficult to differentiate from complicating carcinoma (2–3% of patients).

Glandular calcifications and pan-

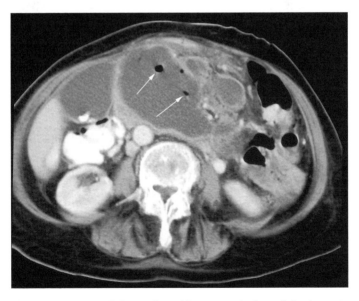

Fig. 7.12 Post-contrast CT in a patient with a pancreatic abscess following acute pancreatitis. There is a fluid collection in relation to the pancreatic body and this contains bubbles of air (small arrows) suggestive of abscess formation. No normal pancreas is seen in this section.

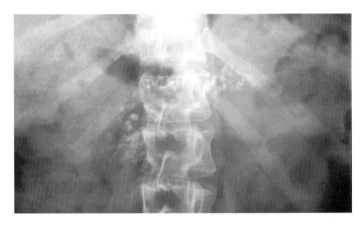

Fig. 7.13 AXR demonstrating pancreatic calcifications in a patient with chronic pancreatitis.

creatic duct dilatation are well demonstrated. Other complications of chronic pancreatitis are visualized (e.g. pseudoaneurysm and splenic vein thrombosis).

ERCP and MRCP

ERCP and, more recently, MRCP are also useful in the diagnosis of chronic pancreatitis. They demonstrate well the changes of dilatation and stricturing that initially involve the side branches and later the main pancreatic duct itself (Fig. 7.14).

Pancreatic carcinoma

Ductal adenocarcinoma is the most common form and occurs usually in the pancreatic head. Presenting symptoms of pancreatic carcinoma are often non-specific but include pain radiating to the back and weight loss. Patients with tumours in the head may present with painless obstructive jaundice. Accurate imaging is required to determine the presence and operability of a tumour.

US

US is usually requested for initial assessment of epigastric pain or jaundice. It is accurate in evaluation of the biliary tree, hepatic parenchyma and ascites, and will often demonstrate a pancreatic mass.

CT

CT, however, is the modality of choice for suspected pancreatic malignancy. CT will usually demonstrate the pancreatic

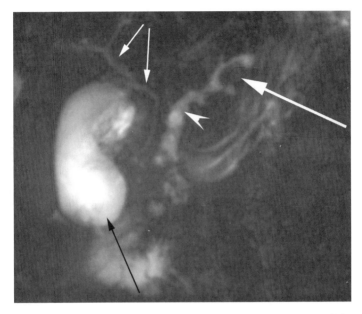

Fig. 7.14 Image from a T2-weighted MRCP sequence. There is dilatation of the pancreatic duct (arrowhead), with clubbed dilated side-branches. A low signal calculus is seen in the pancreatic duct (large white arrow). Note normal common bile duct (small white arrows) and gall bladder (black arrow).

mass (Fig. 7.15) and features that make it unresectable:

• Venous or arterial encasement by tumour
• Invasion of local structures
• Nodal or mesenteric involvement by tumour
• Hepatic or lung metastases.

MR

MR has also proved useful in tumour detection and staging. Its use is generally reserved for cases equivocal at CT.

ERCP

This is particularly useful when other imaging modalities have demonstrated duct dilatation, but no definite cause (Fig. 7.16).

Histological confirmation of malignancy can be obtained by US- or CT-guided aspiration or biopsy of the pancreatic lesion if accessible, or at ERCP.

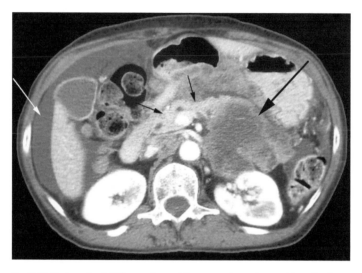

Fig. 7.15 Post-contrast CT in a patient with pancreatic carcinoma. There is a large hypodense mass in the pancreatic tail (large black arrow). The splenic vein has been invaded and is not seen. Normal pancreatic head and body are indicated by small black arrows. Ascites is present (white arrow).

Bile duct stricture

Patients may present with right upper quadrant pain, jaundice and symptoms of malignancy if a malignant aetiology.

Strictures may be:
• *Benign:* iatrogenic is the most common (e.g. post-laparoscopic cholecystectomy)
• *Malignant:* cholangiocarcinoma, carcinoma of gall bladder or pancreas, compression by adjacent nodes.

US

US is accurate in the evaluation of intrahepatic and common bile duct dilata-

tion. It may also demonstrate focal lesions relating to gall bladder, porta hepatis or pancreas.

CT

CT is used for further assessment if US confirms duct dilatation and/or suspected malignancy. As CT is not affected by patient size or bowel gas, it often provides additional information concerning level and cause of duct obstruction and nodal status.

ERCP and PTC

ERCP or percutaneous transhepatic cholangiography (PTC) often represent

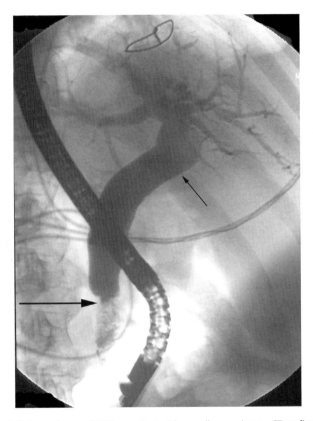

Fig. 7.16 Image from an ERCP in a patient with ampullary carcinoma. CT confirmed dilated ducts, but no obvious cause. ERCP demonstrates a dilated common bile duct (small arrow) and a shouldered stricture at the ampulla (large arrow). Biopsy at ERCP confirmed carcinoma.

the next diagnostic and therapeutic step. PTC is useful if ERCP fails or when pathology may be better treated percutaneously (e.g. mass at hilum of liver). At PTC the liver is punctured and a dilated duct entered, often using US guidance. A drain can be passed via this route to decompress the biliary tree and through it strictures can be traversed using guidewires, dilated by balloon catheter, or a stent deployed (Figs 7.17 & 7.18). Adequate patient preparation is essential (Table 7.1). Biliary leaks and sepsis are additional complications of PTC and antibiotic prophylaxis is usually indicated.

Abdominal trauma

Trauma is the most common cause of death in young adults. Car accidents, falls and assault are the most frequent

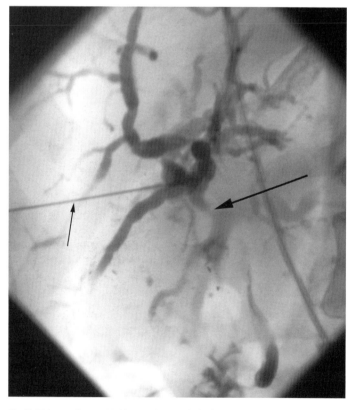

Fig. 7.17 Image from a PTC in a patient with cholangiocarcinoma of the common hepatic duct. Puncture needle is demonstrated (small arrow). There is dilatation of the intrahepatic ducts down to the confluence with a stricture seen involving the upper common bile duct (large arrow).

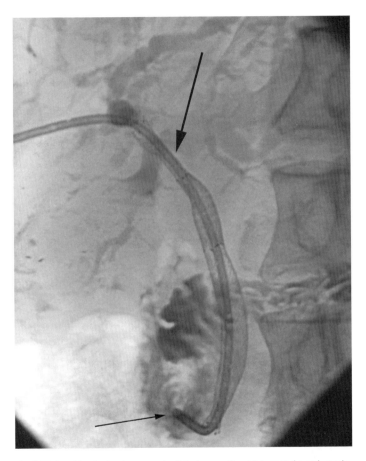

Fig. 7.18 A guidewire has been manipulated across the stricture and a catheter introduced with its tip in the duodenum (small arrow). A self-expanding metallic stent has been introduced to lie across the stricture—note stent 'waisting' (large arrow).

causes of major blunt abdominal trauma. Clinical assessment of abdominal trauma is often unreliable. Resuscitation and stabilization should be undertaken prior to imaging.

Radiography

The basic initial major trauma series of radiographs includes films of chest, cervical spine, abdomen and pelvis. AXR is insensitive in detecting free intra-abdominal fluid, but may demonstrate associated fractures in pelvis, spine or ribs.

US

US has limitations in evaluation of major abdominal trauma. Because of associated wounds and fractures, bandaging, patient discomfort and often large amounts of bowel gas, accurate visualization of intra-abdominal organs is frequently impossible. US will miss many liver, splenic and renal injuries and most pancreatic and bowel injuries.

US does detect free peritoneal fluid and can assess the presence of haemoperitoneum in unstable patients,

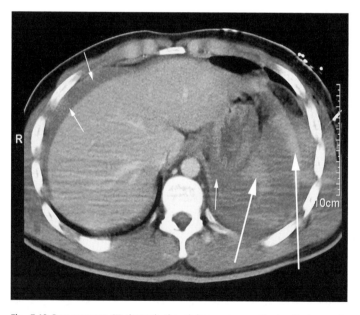

Fig. 7.19 Post-contrast CT through the abdomen in a patient with traumatic splenic rupture with only fragments of enhancing spleen identified (large arrows). Haemoperitoneum is present (small arrows). Streak image artefacts are secondary to monitor leads.

reducing the need for diagnostic peritoneal lavage.

In many cases, if the patient is unstable with evidence of abdominal injury, peritoneal lavage will confirm haemoperitoneum and the patient will transfer to theatre.

CT

If patients can be haemodynamically stabilized, CT is the imaging modality of choice for assessment of the abdomen and pelvis. If patients are to be transferred to CT then it is essential they are stable, with established venous access and medical accompaniment.

Effective CT significantly reduces the incidence of negative laparotomy. It can also provide reassurance where physical examination is difficult (e.g. coexisting head trauma, intoxication).

CT accurately demonstrates haemoperitoneum. CT also has a high degree of accuracy in visualizing hepatic, splenic and renal injuries. The extent of laceration and associated splenic haematoma can be graded (Fig. 7.19) and up to 50% of adults with splenic injury avoid surgery. The majority of hepatic and renal injuries in haemodynamically stable patients are also managed conservatively (Fig. 7.20). In patients treated non-operatively, CT is

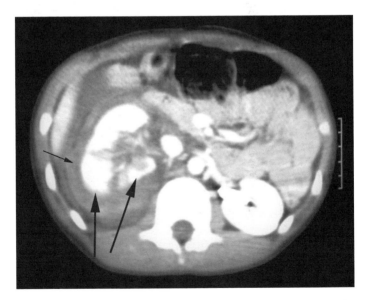

Fig. 7.20 Post-contrast CT demonstrates a fractured right kidney post-trauma. The kidney is fragmented (large arrows) but is perfused, suggesting the vascular pedicle is not damaged. Note extensive perirenal haematoma (small arrow).

used for follow-up to confirm resolution of haemoperitoneum and healing of lacerations.

CT can also diagnose injuries to mesentery and bowel. Free intraperitoneal air, bowel wall thickening and fluid between bowel loops are signs of bowel injury.

Other modalities

IVU and other contrast studies are rarely indicated. Stable patients with microscopic haematuria only do not usually need further investigation.

Angiography is rarely used but may be indicated in some cases of vascular injury and coil embolization can be used to treat active extravasation from a damaged vessel.

Further reading

Gore RM, Levine MS, eds. *Textbook of Gastrointestinal Radiology*, 2nd edn. Philadelphia: Saunders, 2000.

Levine MS, Rubesin SE, Laufer I, eds. *Double Contrast Gastrointestinal Radiology*, 3rd edn. Philadelphia: Saunders, 2000.

Miller FH, ed. *The Radiological Clinics of North America: Radiology of the Pancreas, Gall bladder and Biliary Tract*, Vol. 40. 2002.

Chapter 8: **The breast**

This chapter covers:
Common conditions
- Benign disease: cysts, fibroadenoma, inflammatory disease
- Malignant disease

Common presentations in which imaging can help
- Patients with symptomatic breast disease are those who present with abnormalities they have detected themselves. The NHS, as in many countries, runs a breast screening programme for women who are asymptomatic and the imaging techniques are common to both groups
- This section will relate to the symptomatic breast
- Most patients will present with a lump or area of nodularity. Other symptoms include breast pain (mastalgia) or nipple discharge
- If clinical examination reveals an area of concern, eg. lump, bloody (ie non-physiological) nipple discharge, asymmetric pain of recent onset, axillary adenopathy then the patient should be referred for imaging
- Preferably, patients will attend a joint or multidisciplinary clinic where the surgeon, radiologist and pathologist work together to gain a diagnosis as quickly as possible

Imaging strategy

The two principal imaging modalities used in initial symptomatic breast assessment are mammography and US. Which modality is used depends on the patient's age and the problem to be investigated. The two techniques are complementary and are often used together.

Patients often need to undergo fine needle aspiration for cytology. It should be recognized that this will interfere with the image appearances of a mass lesion and make interpretation difficult if not impossible. However, delays in diagnosis should be avoided.

Mammography

This involves the use of ionizing radiation with radiographs of each breast performed in two planes: lateral oblique and craniocaudal (obl or CC labels on the film). The equipment and film used are specific to mammography and there is a small radiation dose. High-quality imaging is essential to make reliable diagnoses. Do not rely on poor-quality images.

Because of the radiation dose, mammography is not used routinely in young or pregnant patients and it may not be technically feasible in the elderly, infirm or those with extreme breast tenderness (e.g. breast abscess).

Mammography is accurate at demonstrating mass lesions in the breast, can characterize them to some extent and is the technique of choice for detection of malignant microcalcifications. The sensitivity of mammography is significantly reduced in young women with dense glandular breasts.

US

US is non-invasive and does not involve the use of ionizing radiation. It is not used as a screening tool but is used in areas of palpable abnormality, often complementing mammography. It is useful in further characterization of opacities seen mammographically (cyst or solid) and also a useful adjunct in the mammographically dense breast where focal lesions may be obscured.

US is often the only imaging modality utilized in young and pregnant patients. It is used to guide fine needle aspiration or core biopsy of breast lesions and to examine the liver for metastatic spread.

Other modalities

NM

Scintigraphy is used as a second-line investigation in some high-risk patients for detection of additional malignant lesions and for regional nodal assessment. Bone scintigraphy is valuable for patients with suspected bony metastatic disease.

MR

MR is useful for implant assessment and assessment of possible tumour recurrence.

CT

CT is not used for primary diagnosis but is used widely for staging of malignant disease and monitoring its progress.

Benign breast disease

Cysts

Cysts are a common cause of a palpable breast lump. In young women, clinical cysts may be aspirated in clinic and no imaging is required. Many patients undergo mammography and US for further assessment.

Mammography may demonstrate a circumscribed opacity (Fig. 8.1). US is almost 100% accurate in simple cyst characterization (Fig. 8.2). Many cysts are complex, however, following instrumentation or haemorrhage and require further investigation (either by follow-up US or aspiration).

Fibroadenoma

Fibroadenoma is the most common benign breast tumour, usually occurring in young women.

US may be the only modality utilized in patients <30 years and will demonstrate a circumscribed solid nodule (Fig. 8.3). US can guide aspiration or biopsy for confirmation.

Mammography may demonstrate a well-circumscribed opacity and US is used for further characterization.

Breast inflammatory disease

Breast inflammatory disease usually occurs postpartum, during lactation. US is useful if abscess formation is

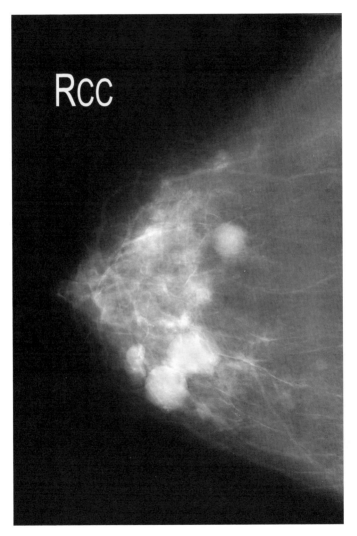

Fig. 8.1 Craniocaudal mammogram of the right breast in a patient with multiple circumscribed breast opacities. These are consistent with cysts and US would confirm this. For orientation of a craniocaudal mammogram, imagine you are looking down at the breast towards the patient's feet and radiographical markers are placed in the axilla (laterally).

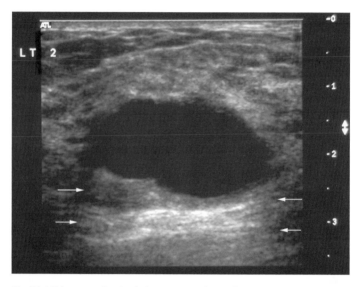

Fig. 8.2 US features of a simple breast cyst: a thin-walled anechoic structure with associated distal acoustic enhancement (arrows) caused by through-transmission of sound through fluid.

suspected clinically. Mammography is not usually performed in acute inflammation because of pain from compression.

Breast carcinoma

Ductal carcinoma is the most common histological subtype and may be preceded by ductal carcinoma *in situ* (DCIS). DCIS may manifest itself mammographically as ductal microcalcification (Fig. 8.4).

Carcinoma usually presents as a palpable lump in the symptomatic breast, although pain, bloody nipple discharge or nipple rash (Paget's disease) may also occur. Further evaluation includes mammography, usually US, and also fine needle aspiration or biopsy.

Mammography

Mammographical features to look for are (Fig. 8.5):
• Ill-defined or spiculated mass
• Parenchymal distortion
• Overlying skin thickening
• Malignant microcalcifications
• Enlarged axillary lymph nodes.

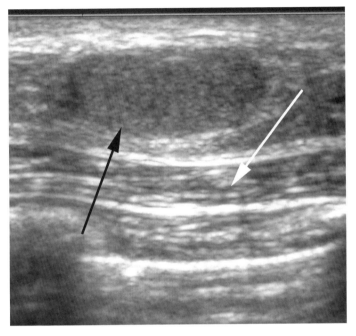

Fig. 8.3 US of a fibroadenoma: an elliptical circumscribed solid nodule (black arrow). Note distal acoustic enhancement and underlying pectoral muscle (white arrow).

US

US features to look for are (Fig. 8.6):
- Ill-defined, usually hypoechoic mass
- Distal acoustic shadowing (caused by sound distortion and diffraction by tumour)
- Surrounding halo—caused by oedema or tumour infiltration
- Abnormal axillary nodes.

Metastases

CXR is used in initial staging for lung or rib metastases. In patients with aggressive tumours at risk of metastases or those with clinical evidence of metastatic disease, further investigation is indicated. This will concentrate on the liver (US or CT) and bones (X-ray of affected area and bone scintigraphy). MR can be useful in patients with equivocal bone scintigraphy.

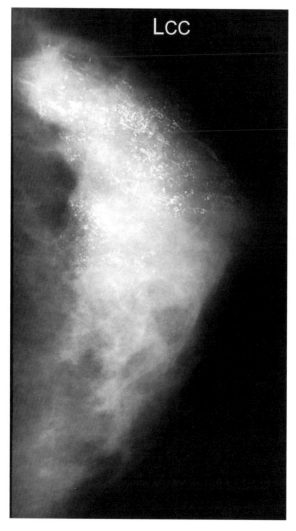

Fig. 8.4 Left craniocaudal mammogram of DCIS: extensive malignant-type calcifications are seen within the outer breast. They are branching (following ducts) and differ in size, shape and density. This patient is young; note how dense the breast parenchyma is.

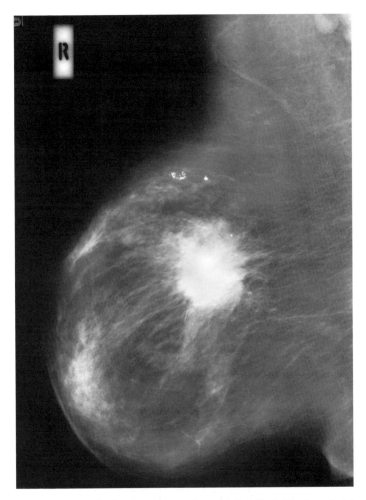

Fig. 8.5 Right lateral oblique mammogram in an elderly patient with a large ductal carcinoma. This mass is ill-defined and spicules extend widely into the surrounding breast. The spicules can relate to tumour infiltration or inflammation. The breast generally is far more lucent than the patient in Fig. 8.4; fatty replacement of dense glandular tissue is occurring. Some benign calcifications are also present in the breast.

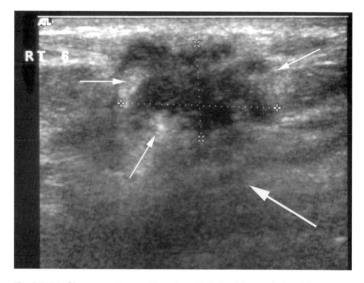

Fig. 8.6 US of breast carcinoma. There is an ill-defined hypoechoic solid mass (callipers). Note hyperechoic halo surrounding (small white arrows). There is some distal acoustic shadowing (large white arrow).

Further reading

Feig SA, ed. *Radiological Clinics of North America: Breast Imaging* 2000; Vol. 38 (4).

Howlett DC, Marchbank NDP, Allan SM. Sonographic assessment of the symptomatic breast. *Journal of Diagnostic Radiography and Imaging* 2003; **5**: 1–10.

Chapter 9: **Musculoskeletal system**

This chapter covers:
Common conditions
- Osteoarthritis, rheumatoid arthritis, gout
- Metastases, myeloma
- The cervical spine: trauma and rheumatoid arthritis
- Osteoporosis
- Colles' fracture, femoral neck fractures
- Infection: osteomyelitis, septic arthritis
- Other conditions: diabetic foot, Paget's disease

Common presentations in which imaging can help
- Pain: most musculoskeletal conditions
- Swelling: often in joints
- Sepsis: septic arthritis, osteomyelitis
- Systemic illness (e.g. weight loss, malaise): metastatic disease, myeloma, rheumatoid arthritis

Imaging strategy

With the wide range of imaging modalities available, all of which can give valuable information, a rational evidence-based approach to imaging is crucial.

Radiography

The plain radiograph should be the first investigation in most circumstances.

Correctly positioned radiographs in two orthogonal planes are desirable, particularly in trauma: these are usually an AP view and a lateral projection. Inclusion of the entire anatomical part and the relevant joints will help to avoid missed diagnoses. Do not forget referred pain and paraesthesiae! Comparison with previous radiographs is often extremely helpful in evaluating the significance of the imaging findings. Plain film findings in musculoskeletal disorders are often subtle, and liaison with a radiologist will help to focus the imaging pathway for each individual patient.

NM

NM is often utilized early in the investigation of musculoskeletal conditions, with a particular role in the evaluation of suspected metastatic disease, infection and occult fractures.

CT

CT is used for further assessment of some fractures, particularly in the cervical region, and can also be used to guide bone biopsy procedures.

MR

MR is an excellent modality for non-invasive imaging of bones, joints and soft tissues generally. It is extremely useful in a problem-solving role. In general, CT is good for looking at bone changes, whereas MR is more sensitive in demonstrating soft-tissue changes and excess fluid (e.g. in joints).

US

US is useful at evaluating superficial soft tissues and tendons, and also for demonstrating and aspirating joint effusions.

Osteoarthritis

This is the most common disorder of the joints in the adult. It is more common in weight-bearing joints, but all the joints may be affected. Cartilage breakdown is the underlying pathological process.

The general radiological appearances include (Fig. 9.1):
• Loss of joint space as a result of breakdown in the joint cartilage. This tends to be greatest in the areas exposed to the greatest load and therefore may be asymmetrical.
• Subchondral bony sclerosis occurs as new bone formation develops.
• Osteophyte formation at the margins of the joint is seen.
• Subchondral cysts or geodes form at areas of stress on articular cartilage and subchondral bone.

The radiological features at specific joints are as follow:
• *The hands and feet:*
  – More frequent in older patients and much more common in women
  – Metacarpophalangeal and carpometacarpal joint of the thumb and the carpal joints of the radial side of the carpus are very commonly affected
  – Distal interphalangeal joint osteophytosis in the hands is clinically described as Heberden's nodes and within the proximal interphalangeal joints is called Bouchard's nodes
  – Metatarsophalangeal joint of the great toe is commonly involved.
• *The knee:*
  – The most commonly involved joint
  – Medial tibiofemoral and patellofemoral compartments are most commonly involved, which can lead to varus deformity
  – Osteophyte formation leds to peaking of the tibial spines
  – Bony fragments may be present as loose bodies.
• *The hip* (Fig. 9.1):
  – Joint space narrowing is most often seen superiorly within the joint, with superior and lateral displacement of the femoral head
  – Cortical thickening or buttressing of the femoral neck may be seen.
• *The spine:*
  – Degenerative change at the insertion of the annulus fibrosus leads to osteophyte formation along the margins of the vertebral end plates, which may extend to the adjacent end plate—bridging osteophytosis
  – Loss of disc hydration within the nucleus pulposus leads to loss of disc height
  – Degenerative change can be seen within the apophyseal joints and the costovertebral joints with hypertrophic osteophyte formation.

Rheumatoid arthritis

Rheumatoid arthritis is the most common adult connective tissue disorder. It is a symmetrical inflammatory polyarthropathy with a predilection for

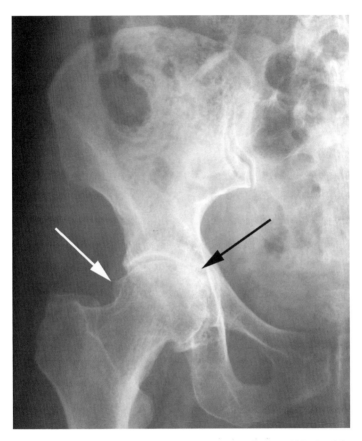

Fig. 9.1 This AP radiograph demonstrates degenerative change within the right hip joint. Osteophytosis (white arrow) with geode formation (black arrow) is noted within the right hip joint with loss of joint space medially.

the small joints of the hands and feet. Larger joints such as the shoulder, elbow, hip, knee and ankle can be affected.

Diagnostic criteria require at least four of the following to be present:

- Morning stiffness
- Swelling of three or more joints, especially the wrist, metatarsophalangeal or proximal interphalangeal joints, for more than 6 weeks

- Symmetrical swelling
- Typical radiographical changes
- Rheumatoid nodules
- Positive rheumatoid factor.

Radiographs of the hands and feet should be obtained in the first instance. In the hands and wrists, the changes are commonly seen within metacarpopha-langeal joints, proximal interphalangeal joints, intercarpal joints, ulnar styloid and distal radio-ulnar joint. The metatarsophalangeal joints and inter-

phalangeal joints of the feet are com-monly affected early in the disease.

The early plain film appearances include (Fig. 9.2):
- Fusiform periarticular soft-tissue swelling (joint effusion)
- Periarticular, then diffuse osteopenia
- Widened joint space
- Marginal bone erosions
- Erosion of ulnar styloid.

The later plain film appearances include:

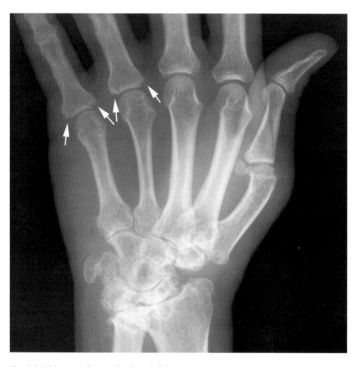

Fig. 9.2 This AP radiograph of the left hand demonstrates periarticular osteopenia at the metacarpophalangeal joints with periarticular erosive changes in associa-tion (white arrows). Note erosive and secondary degenerative changes also present in the corpus with erosion of the ulnar styloid process.

• Diffuse loss of joint space from cartilage loss
• Flexion and extension contractions with ulnar subluxation and dislocation
• Marked destruction of the articular surface of joints
• Destruction of bone ends.

CXR may demonstrate resorption of distal ends of clavicles with upward displacement of humeral heads resulting from tear or atrophy of the supraspinatous muscle and tendon. Pulmonary soft-tissue masses (rheumatoid nodules) may be seen on the plain film. The pelvic radiograph may demonstrate protusio acetabuli with migration of the femoral head into the acetabulum and ileum. Atlanto-axial subluxation within the cervical spine is important to recognize (see later in this chapter).

Useful differentiating features of rheumatoid arthritis from other arthropathies are:
• The erosive changes in rheumatoid arthritis are rarely associated with hypertrophic bone changes such as sclerosis, spurs or periosteal reaction
• The distribution is symmetrical with diffuse uniform cartilage loss
• Erosive changes are most severe within the hands and feet
• Involvement of larger joints is late in the disease process
• The thoracic and lumbar spine are usually spared
• Sclerosis of the sacroiliac joints with erosions is rarely found.

Gout

Primary gout is an inborn error of purine metabolism associated with hyperuricaemia and recurrent episodes of acute arthritis. Men are much more commonly affected than women. Secondary gout is associated with myeloproliferative disorders and their treatment, blood dyscrasias and chronic renal failure.

The affected joint is acutely painful, hot and swollen. This is classically within the metatarsophalangeal joint of the great toe. The plain film demonstrates soft-tissue swelling and joint effusion. The main differential diagnosis is acute septic arthritis.

Chronic tophaceous gout occurs 5–10 years after the first initial attack. This develops in half of the patients with recurrent acute gout. Early treatment may delay the development of bony lesions.

The plain film appearances of chronic tophaceous gout include (Fig. 9.3):
• Nodular deposition of calcium monosodium urate crystals (tophi) may be within the synovium, subchondral bone (Fig. 9.3), helix of the ear and soft tissues of the hand, elbow, foot, knee and forearm. These may calcify.
• Chondrocalcinosis, especially within the soft tissues of the knee.
• Bony erosions (Fig. 9.3) may be intraarticular, periarticular or distant from the joint.
• The classic X-ray appearance is of a round or oval erosion with sclerotic margins and an overhanging margin of bone (Fig. 9.3).

Important differentiating features from other arthropathies:
• Gout is asymmetrical
• There is little or no osteopenia until late in the disease
• The joint space is preserved until late.

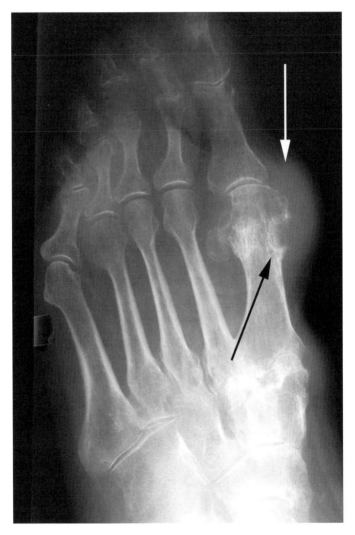

Fig. 9.3 This radiograph demonstrates a rounded soft-tissue mass overlying the metatarsophalangeal joint of the great toe (white arrow). There is a well-defined erosion of the head of the metatarsal of the great toe, with sclerotic overhanging margins characteristic of gouty arthropathy (black arrow).

Skeletal metastases

Carcinomatous metastases are by far the most common malignancy of the skeleton. The clinical presentation is of bony pain or pathological fracture. Metastasis should always be considered in symptomatic patients with a known history of primary tumour. Fracture secondary to minimal trauma should also raise the suspicion of pathological fracture. Most metastases to bone are osteolytic. Sclerotic or mixed appearances do occur but less commonly. Sclerosis after chemotherapy is recognized.

Lytic metastases

These most commonly arise from carcinoma of the breast, bronchus, kidney, uterus and gastrointestinal tract, but do not forget lymphoma. The site of involvement may vary but the axial skeleton, the spine, skull, pelvis and proximal long bones are most commonly affected. If you encounter metastasis in the smaller bones, then think of carcinoma of the bronchus, breast and kidney first.

The radiological features of lytic metastases are:
• They are often multiple.
• They have poorly defined margins within the medulla of bone. (Evaluation of the margin of a lytic lesion on the plain radiograph is extremely useful in deciding whether it is a benign or malignant lesion—if in doubt, ask a radiologist).
• Lytic lesions after chemotherapy or radiotherapy may become sclerotic. A careful history is therefore important.
• Ill-defined cortical destruction with extension into the soft tissues.

• Bony expansion is unusual but may be seen in carcinoma of the kidney and thyroid (Fig. 9.4).

Pathological fracture should always be considered when:
• There is a history of a known carcinoma
• The fracture margins are ill defined and irregular
• The underlying medullary and cortical bone demonstrates ill-defined lytic lesions or destructive changes
• The trauma was minimal.

Sclerotic metastases

Prostatic carcinoma is the most common cause (see Chapter 11, Fig. 11.13), but carcinoma of the breast, gastrointestinal tract, bladder and cervix may produce sclerotic metastasis.

Radiological appearances on the plain film include:
• Patchy sclerosis with loss of the normal corticomedullary appearances
• Extension through the cortex with ill-defined periosteal reaction
• Some lytic destructive elements
• Comparison with previous films and careful history may help in differentiating Paget's disease from sclerotic metastasis.

Some important things to remember in the radiological assessment of metastases

• The initial plain X-ray obtained may be normal.
• In cases of strong clinical concern, especially in patients with known primary tumour, further evaluation with isotope bone scanning should be undertaken (Fig. 9.5). This has a significantly higher sensitivity than plain radiography.

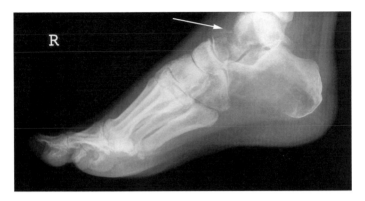

Fig. 9.4 This is a lateral radiograph of the right foot in a patient with metastatic renal cell carcinoma. There is a large and ill-defined lytic lesion in the calcaneum also involving adjacent talus and cuboid. Complete destruction of the inferior calcaneal cortex can be seen. There is a pathological fracture of the neck of the talus with ill-defined margins in keeping with pathological fracture (arrow).

• An MR examination may be a better alternative in patients with suspected spinal metastasis, especially if there is coexistent degenerative change within the spine, and should be considered in cases with neurological manifestations combined with spinal pain.
• MRI is helpful in patients with osteoporosis and vertebral crush fractures with suspected spinal metastasis.
• A radiologist's opinion is valuable.

Myeloma

Myeloma is the most common primary malignant bone neoplasm in adults and represents a malignant proliferation of plasma cells.

Clinical features include:
• Peak incidence range is 50–80 years of age

• Twice as common in males
• Presentation with bone pain in 60–70% of cases
• Anaemia, which is normochromic and normocytic
• Bence Jones proteinaemia with monoclonal gammopathy
• Hypercalcaemia
• Renal insufficiency.
 Radiological features on the plain film are:
• *Small well-defined 'punched-out' lytic lesions:* throughout the skeleton, often involving the skull (Fig. 9.6)
• *Generalized osteopenia:* this may mimic osteoporosis, but generalized osteopenia in men in their fifties and sixties should raise suspicion of myeloma as osteoporosis in this group is rare
• *Pathological fracture:* this affects half of these patients and is most commonly a vertebral compression fracture.

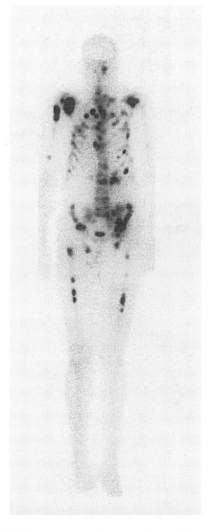

Fig. 9.5 Whole body isotope bone scan demonstrating multiple pathological areas of isotope uptake throughout the skeleton in keeping with disseminated skeletal metastases.

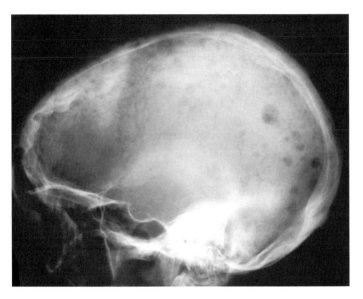

Fig. 9.6 Multiple 'punched out' lytic lesions can be seen throughout the calvarium, which are typical of myelomatous bony involvement.

Sclerosis may be seen within lesions after radiotherapy. Isotope bone scan may be negative in 25–50% of lesions as these do not demonstrate increased isotope uptake.

The cervical spine

Cervical spine radiographs are routinely performed as part of a trauma series and initial immobilization of the cervical spine is essential. The cervical spine should not be mobilized until radiological and clinical evaluation has excluded a fracture. Cervical spine films are also requested for the investigation of neck pain and for symptoms referred to the arms and legs.

The number of radiographical views obtained in trauma depends on the patient's condition. The single most important projection is the lateral view. Ensure all seven cervical bodies are visualized and the C7/T1 junction is seen (fracture dislocation may occur at this level). If the patient's condition permits, an AP view and an open mouth odontoid view should be obtained. If the entire cervical spine with C7/T1 junction is not visualized then ask the radiographer whether a 'swimmer's view' is possible, considering the patient's condition. The alternative is a CT scan of the nonvisualized cervical spine. If a fracture is demonstrated on plain radiographs then CT may be indicated for further evaluation. Patients with associated neurological abnormalities may need to be evaluated with MR. Ask a radiologist.

In viewing the lateral radiograph of the cervical spine, it is important to assess the bony structures and to assess the alignment of the vertebral bodies. Each vertebral body together with its posterior elements should be evaluated carefully. Loss of vertebral body height, depression of the vertebral end plates or discontinuity in the cortical outline of the vertebral bodies and the posterior elements may indicate fracture. Normally, the intervertebral discs are symmetrical in appearance, without loss of height or localized asymmetrical widening or narrowing. Following trauma, assessment of alignment and articulation is critical. The relationship of the various structures can be assessed using anatomical landmarks and imaginary 'lines' superimposed on the lateral radiograph. These are demonstrated in Fig. 9.7. If in doubt, seek the view of a radiologist.

Acute cervical spine trauma

A full and complete description of all possible cervical fractures and trauma is beyond the scope of this chapter. A brief review of the main types of fracture that may be encountered is presented. The crucial thing is to decide whether a fracture is stable or unstable. Unstable fractures may require urgent surgical intervention and specialist referral is essential. If there is any clinical doubt, then it is always wise to seek an experienced specialist opinion as soon as possible.

The classification of cervical fractures is related to the mechanism of injury. The patterns of injury include hyperflexion, hyperextension, vertical compression, flexion–rotation and lateral flexion (shearing) injuries.

Hyperflexion injury

These are the most common injuries of the cervical spine, including the 'whiplash injury'. These are usually associated with ligamentous disruption of the posterior ligaments.
- *Flexion 'teardrop' fracture:*
  – Unstable.
  – There is often severe neurological deficit below the level of fracture associated with quadriplegia.
  – Lateral view demonstrates localized flexion of the cervical spine with a bony fragment ('teardrop') representing a fracture of the antero-inferior part of the vertebral body. Vertebral body subluxation and widening of the facet joints is associated.
- *Simple wedge fracture and clay shoveller's fracture* (Fig. 9.8): fractures of the spinous process, most commonly C6/7 or T1 are stable.
- *Anterior subluxation:* may be stable initially but can become unstable as a result of incomplete ligamentous healing. Look for forward vertebral body subluxation associated with localized forward flexion.
- *Bilateral facetal dislocation:* an unstable injury associated with forward vertebral body subluxation and dislocation of both facet joints of the affected vertebral body.

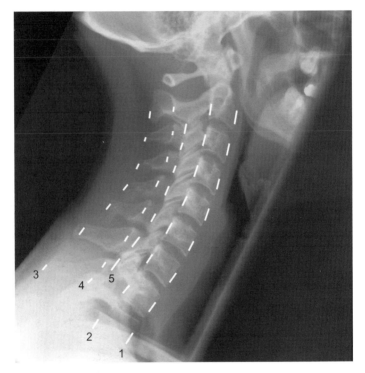

Fig. 9.7 Normal lateral cervical spine radiograph. The 'imaginary' lines are demonstrated.
1 The anterior longitudinal line joins the anterior margins of the junction of the spinous process and lamina.
2 The posterior longitudinal line runs along the posterior vertebral bodies.
3 The spinous line connects the tips of the spinous processes.
4 The spinolaminar line joins the anterior margins of the junction of the spinous process and lamina.
5 The posterior pillar line connects the posterior surface of the articular pillars.
The laminar space lies between the spinolaminar line (4) and the posterior pillar line (5).

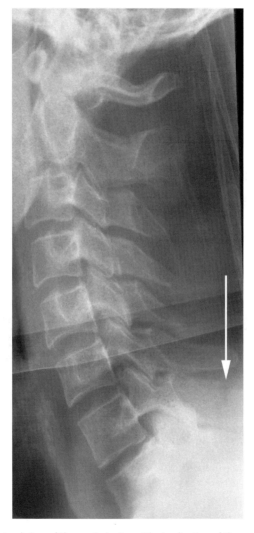

Fig. 9.8 Lateral view of the cervical spine with visualization of the cervical spine down to C7/T1. There is a fracture of the spinous process of C7 (arrow). This is called a clay shoveller's fracture.

Hyperextension injury

• *The 'hangman's fracture':* an unstable fracture of both neural arches of C2 associated with prevertebral soft-tissue swelling, forward slip of C2 on C3 and fracture of the antero-inferior tip of C2.

• *'Teardrop' fracture associated with extension:* an unstable injury involving a fracture of the antero-inferior tip of the effected vertebral body, usually C2.

Vertical compression injury

• *Jefferson fracture* (Fig. 9.9a,b): an unstable injury with fractures of the anterior and posterior arches of C1. This is caused by axial force applied to the skull with impaction of the occipital condyles onto the lateral masses of C1. An AP or open mouth view may demonstrate lateral displacement of the lateral masses of C1.

• *Burst fracture:* caused by an axial force causing impaction of the intervertebral disc into the vertebral end plate below with a comminuted fracture of the vertebral body below. Fracture fragments may displace into the spinal canal. CT is helpful in demonstrating these.

The cervical spine in rheumatoid arthritis

The atlanto-axial joint is the most common site of rheumatoid involvement within the spine. Atlanto-axial subluxation occurs in up to 6% of patients with rheumatoid arthritis and is demonstrated as an increase in distance between the posterior surface of the anterior arch of C1 and the anterior surface of the dens of >2.5 mm (Fig. 9.10).

This is important in the preoperative assessment of the rheumatoid patient as cervical spine extension associated with intubation may lead to cord compression.

Passive flexion and extension views may be helpful as increasing atlanto-axial space on flexion may indicate atlanto-axial instability.

On the radiographs:

• Look for subluxation of the odontoid on the flexion view

• Look for erosions of the odontoid peg resulting from synovitis of adjacent bursae

• Remember that the combination of erosion and osteopenia predisposes to fracture of the odontoid peg

• Involvement of the apophyseal joints and disc spaces may occur leading to vertebral body subluxations and bone destruction

• Involvement of the cervical inetevertebral discs may lead to disc narrowing and eventual fusion.

Osteoporosis

Osteoporosis is defined as the reduction of overall bone mass. This is a common metabolic disorder in postmenopausal women and the elderly. Other rarer causes of osteoporosis include:

• Drugs: steroids and heparin

• Metabolic conditions: Cushing's disease, hyperthyroidism, hyperparathyroidism, hypogonadism, acromegaly, diabetes mellitus and pregnancy

• Alcoholism

• Chronic liver disease

• Anaemia.

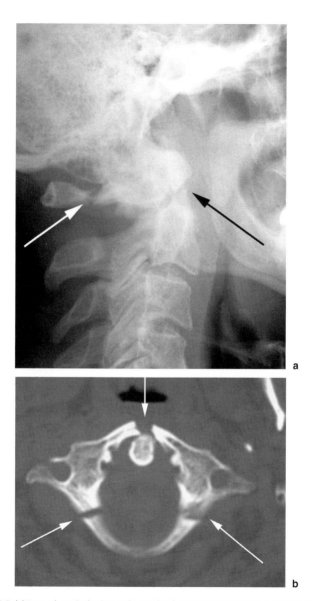

Fig. 9.9 (a) Lateral cervical spine radiograph of a patient involved in a road traffic accident demonstrates fracture of the base of the dens with forward subluxation of C2 in relation to C1 (black arrow). In addition, there is a fracture of the lamina of C1 (white arrow). (b) Axial CT image of C1 demonstrating fractures of the anterior (short white arrow) and posterior arch of C1 (long white arrows).

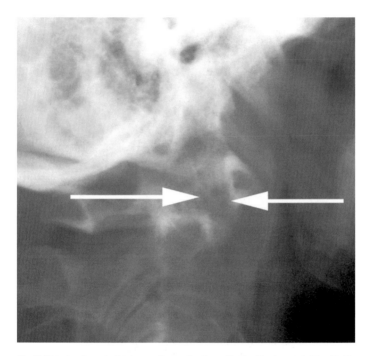

Fig. 9.10 Lateral cervical spine radiograph of a patient with rheumatoid arthritis demonstrates widening of the atlanto-axial space (arrows). Note significant osteopenia within the cervical spine with degenerative changes at multiple levels.

Confirmation of the diagnosis of osteoporosis and follow-up after treatment is most commonly undertaken with dual X-ray absorptiometry (DEXA scanning).

Postmenopausal osteoporosis

Women in the range 50–65 years of age are affected. Excessive loss of trabecular bone occurs, giving rise to rapid bone loss after the menopause. There is an increased incidence of fractures especially the vertebra and distal radius.

Plain film appearances in the spine (Fig. 9.11):
• Radiographs negative until bone loss of 30%
• Decreased overall bone density (osteopenia)

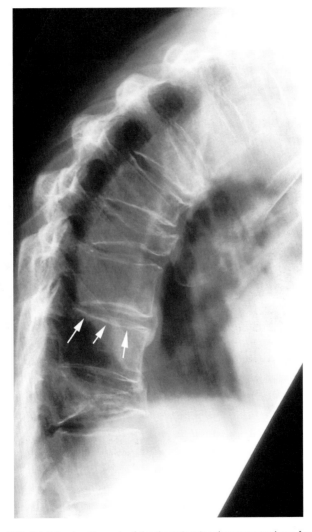

Fig. 9.11 This lateral radiograph of the thoracic spine demonstrates loss of vertebral body height and anterior wedging of several of the thoracic vertebral bodies. This is typical of osteoporotic vertebral body collapse and crush fracture. The bones are generally osteopenic. Note the dense cortical outline of the vertebral bodies demonstrating the typical 'pencilling in' appearance (white arrows).

• Thinning and loss of the secondary horizontal trabecula, with an apparent increase in the primary vertical trabeculae, with subsequent vertical striation appearance to the vertebral body
• The cortices appear thin but dense in relation to the trabecular changes, giving a 'pencilling in' appearance
• Leads to loss of vertebral body height.

Senile osteoporosis

This affects elderly males and females in a ratio of 1 : 2, without having associated accelerated postmenopausal bone loss. There is an increased risk of fractures, most commonly in the femoral neck, proximal humerus, tibia and pelvis. The weakened bones may fracture after only minor trauma.

Insufficiency fractures occur from normal stress on the abnormally weak bones and most commonly affect the sacrum, iliac bones and os pubis. These may not be seen on X-ray. Insufficiency fractures should be suspected in patients with osteoporosis who develop sacral or posterior pelvic pain without a history of trauma. Sacral insufficiency fractures have a characteristic H-shaped pattern of increased isotope uptake on bone scanning. This may help to exclude bony metastasis as the cause.

Other common fractures

Colles' fracture

Colles' fracture is the most common fracture of the forearm and is common in the elderly. It is caused by a fall onto the outstretched hand. Inadequate reduction can lead to post-traumatic arthritis and decreased function. There is distal radial fracture, often with a fracture of the ulnar styloid. Dorsal displacement of the distal fragment gives rise to the 'dinner-fork' deformity.

Plain film appearances are demonstrated in Fig. 9.12.

Fractures of the femoral neck

These are very common and sometimes undiagnosed fractures that occur in elderly patients, particularly women with osteopenia. Any fracture of the femoral neck may lead to disruption of blood supply and to subsequent avascular necrosis of the femoral head.

The following types occur:
• *Subcapital fracture:* at the base of the femoral head. This has a significant incidence of subsequent avascular necrosis of the femoral head.
• *Transcervical fracture:* occurs half way between the femoral head and the intertrochanteric line (Fig. 9.13).
• *Supratrochanteric fracture:* occurs just above the intertrochanteric line.
• *Intertrochanteric fracture:* occurs between the greater and lesser trochanter of the femur.

Osteomyelitis

Osteomyelitis commonly presents with pain, soft-tissue swelling and erythema, inability to weight bear and elevated haematological markers of infection such as a raised white cell count, erythrocyte sedimentation rate (ESR) and C-reactive protein (CRP). Osteomyelitis usually arises from haematogenous spread or from direct contamination in penetrating injuries. The metaphysis of

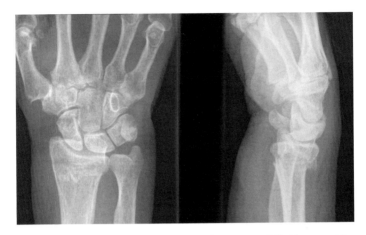

Fig. 9.12 AP and lateral view of the right wrist demonstrates Colles' fracture of the distal radius with angulation.

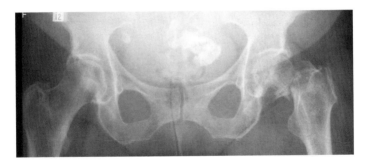

Fig. 9.13 This AP radiograph of both hip joints demonstrates a transcervical fracture of the left neck of femur.

long bones of the lower limbs, vertebrae (lumbar spine is most common) and sacroiliac joints are the most frequent sites of involvement, although small tubular bones in the hands and feet may be affected in diabetes. Diabetes is a significant predisposing condition.

Radiological appearances on plain film:

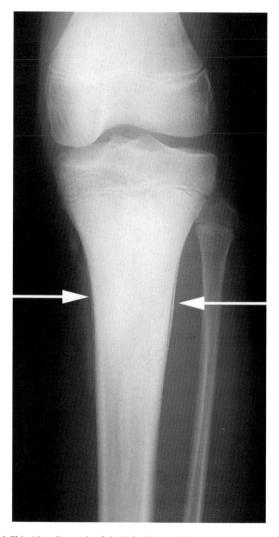

Fig. 9.14 This AP radiograph of the left tibia and fibula demonstrates increased density of the upper tibia with associated periosteal reaction (white arrows) in a patient with osteomyelitis.

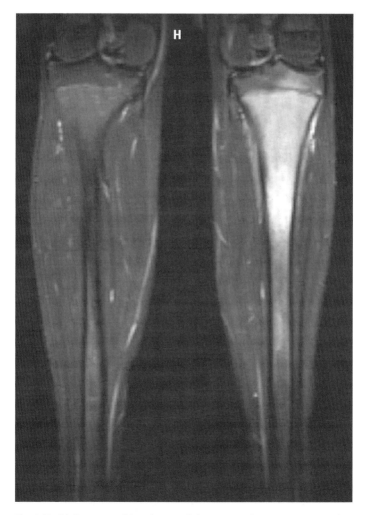

Fig. 9.15 This is a coronal STIR image of the same patient as in Fig. 9.14 (see Chapter 2), which demonstrates extensive marrow high signal (marrow oedema change) within the proximal shaft of the tibia, extending to involve the proximal tibial metaphysis and the lateral aspect of the tibial epiphysis. This MRI examination demonstrates the full extent of involvement.

- Initial radiographs are often normal.
- Early radiological signs are those of soft-tissue swelling and loss of fat planes at 7–10 days.
- Periosteal reaction is usually seen after 2 weeks (Fig. 9.14).
- Ill-defined lytic lesions extend from the metaphysis as infection tracks into the marrow cavity.
- Late signs are areas of detached necrotic cortical bone forming sequestra. These appear as sclerotic areas of bone.
- Pus may extend into the soft tissues.
- Joint involvement is more common in adults than children.
- Left untreated, chronic osteomyelitis, which is characterized by areas of dense sclerotic bone with thickening associated with lucent areas and periosteal reaction, may develop.

Isotope bone scanning and white cell labelled scanning may be used to detect early osteomyelitis, with a sensitivity of 80–90%.

MRI is very sensitive in the early detection of acute osteomyelitis and, unlike NM, does not involve a radiation dose to the patient. The typical features of osteomyelitis on MRI include (Fig. 9.15):

- Low signal intensity within the marrow on T1-weighted images with high signal intensity on T2-weighted and STIR images (see Chapter 2).
- High signal halo surrounding the cortex on T2-weighted images
- Demonstration of bony and soft-tissue abscesses and tracts.

Septic arthritis

Patients with septic arthritis present with a painful, swollen and hot joint with a septic clinical and haematological picture. The hip and knee joints are most commonly involved in children, with the shoulder, sternoclavicular joint, spine, sacroiliac joint and symphysis pubis most common in adults.

Modes of infection:

- Haematogenous spread—particularly in intravenous drug abusers and immunocompromised patients
- As a complication of internal fixation or joint prosthesis
- As a result of direct penetrating injury
- Spread from adjacent osteomyelitis
  Staphylococcus aureus (including MRSA) is the most common organism isolated.

Plain film appearances (Fig. 9.16):

- *Early signs:*
  – Radiographs are initially normal in many cases
  – Soft-tissue swelling with joint effusion.
- *Later signs:* after 1–2 weeks
  – Small ill-defined bony erosions with loss of cortical outline
  – Subchondral bony destruction
  – Areas of reactive sclerosis within the underlying bone.

Early diagnosis and treatment is imperative to avoid permanent joint destruction and ankylosis. US of the hip is helpful in confirming a joint effusion and for guiding aspiration.

The diagnosis is made by obtaining blood cultures and prompt joint aspirate for Gram staining and culture. Radiological guidance is helpful in aspiration of the hip joint, sacroiliac joint and within the spine.

Depending on availability, an isotope bone scan or MR is helpful in cases of clinical doubt.

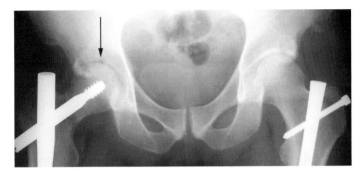

Fig. 9.16 AP radiograph of both hip joints. This patient was involved in a road traffic accident. The patient developed fever with right hip pain. This radiograph demonstrates bilateral internal femoral fixation. There is, in addition, loss of joint space within the right hip joint in comparison with the left, with ill-defined lytic destruction of the acetabular cortex (arrow). The appearances are suspicious for septic arthritis. Aspiration and culture was positive.

Diabetic foot

The diabetic foot is caused by a combination of loss of sensation and proprioception of the affected limb, combined with repetitive trauma. The most common sites affected are the ankle, foot and hand. The clinical presentation is that of a swollen joint, often with deformity, without history of significant trauma, in combination with peripheral neuropathy and loss of proprioception.

The radiological features include (Fig. 9.17):

• Joint effusions in association with soft-tissue swelling.

• Hypertrophic sclerosis of the joints. This affects the subchondral bone and may be rather patchy.

• Atrophic changes with areas of bone resorption, leading to areas of lucency.

• Advanced degenerative changes with bony fragmentation. Subluxation of joints commonly within the mid foot (Charcot's joint).

• Vascular calcification is commonly seen.

• There may be evidence of previous amputation, especially in the feet.

Diagnostic difficulty occurs as many of the above signs also occur with infection. Infection in the feet is a common complication of diabetes and may coexist with the changes based on the peripheral neuropathy described above.

It is important to look for:

• Soft-tissue swelling, with obliteration of the normal fat planes.

• Soft-tissue emphysema seen as small

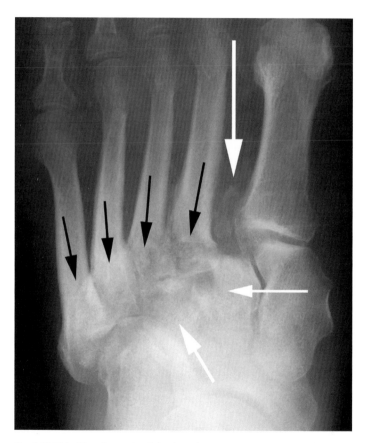

Fig. 9.17 This AP radiograph of the foot demonstrates subluxation of the tarsometatarsal joints of the second, third, fourth and fifth toes (black arrows), with fractures of the bases of the second and third metatarsals, with ill-defined lucency combined with callus formation. Sclerotic change is noted within the middle and lateral cuneiforms (small white arrows) with vascular calcification (large white arrow) present. The appearances are in keeping with diabetes and Charcot's joint.

focal lucencies within the soft tissues. These may be associated with an ulcer, but if the tissue planes distant to an ulcer are affected you must think about anaerobic infection and whether urgent action is required.

• Ill-defined lytic cortical destruction, as this is suggestive of osteomyelitis.

• Periosteal reaction in the absence of fracture.

Comparison with any previous radiographs allows assessment of disease progression and is useful for the subtle changes of early osteomyelitis. A follow-up radiograph after a short interval, with comparison to the initial radiograph, will help in the detection of early infection.

Isotope scanning and MR are extremely useful in the detection of early osteomyelitis and in the evaluation of the extent of involvement.

Paget's disease

British radiologists love Paget's disease as it is uncommon outside Western Europe and has easily recognized radiological features. It is characterized by disordered and exaggerated bone remodelling. It affects the middle-aged and elderly, with increased incidence in men. Geographically common within the UK, it also occurs in Australia, New Zealand and the USA. The axial skele-

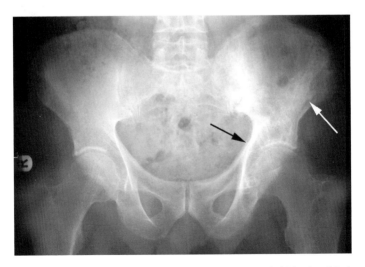

Fig. 9.18 AP radiograph of the pelvis demonstrates cortical thickening (black arrow) within the left hemipelvis, with coarsening of the trabeculae and patchy sclerosis (white arrow) typical for Paget's disease.

ton is the most common site of involvement, affecting the spine (75%), skull (65%), pelvis (40%; Fig. 9.18) and proximal femur (75%).

Ask a radiologist to show you his or her collection! The main point here is that it should not be mistaken for sclerotic metastases, particularly in the pelvis from the prostate, or vice versa. In general, it runs a benign course.

Isotope bone scans are useful in assessing the areas of involvement within the skeleton and this distribution helps to differentiate metastases and can be used in the assessment of disease activity.

Complications of Paget's disease

• *Sarcomatous change and fractures:* if pain occurs in a patient with Paget's disease, think of sarcomatous change— rare, up to 1% of patients overall—and insufficiency fractures of long bones and vertebral compression fractures.

• *Premature osteoarthritis and deformity:* from bowing of long bones and protrusio acetabuli.

• *Neurological complications:* occur in advanced cases due to bone softening and remodelling causing nerve entrapment and cord compression. This may lead to basilar impression and obstructive hydrocephalus.

Further reading

Sutton D, ed. *A Textbook of Radiology and Imaging*, 7th edn. Wangstone, UK: Churchill, 2002.

Chapter 10: **The neck**

This chapter covers:
Common conditions
• Thyroid: benign nodule, goitre, malignancy, thyroiditis
• Salivary gland: sialolithiasis, sialadenitis, tumour
• Cervical adenopathy
Common presentations in which imaging can help
• Palpable mass: thyroid or salivary gland neoplasm, cervical node
• Pain with or without swelling: thyroid or salivary gland malignancy, thyroiditis, sialadenitis
• Systemic illness: metastatic thyroid or salivary gland malignancy, thyroid dysfunction, malignant adenopathy

Imaging strategy

US

US is the initial imaging technique for the investigation of neck diseases. It is readily available, inexpensive, non-invasive and does not involve ionizing radiation. It quickly and accurately distinguishes solid from cystic lesions, can identify additional non-palpable nodules and can be used to guide fine needle aspiration cytology (FNAC). The thyroid, parotid and submandibular glands, and cervical lymph nodes are superficial in location and are readily accessible to high-resolution US examination. US has high accuracy in the detection of salivary gland calculi, associated ductal dilatation and complications such as abscess or sialocele formation. It is effective in salivary gland tumour localization, although it may not be able to delineate the entire extent of very large or deep tumours. US is the first-line investigation of choice in the evaluation of cervical lymphadenopathy, with high sensitivity and specificity, especially when combined with FNAC.

Conventional sialography

Conventional sialography is an invasive procedure that involves duct cannulation, contrast injection and irradiation. It may be required to demonstrate very small calculi, ductal strictures and sialectasis.

It is increasingly being replaced by US and MR sialography, which provide non-invasive assessment of ductal obstruction.

NM

NM provides functional imaging that complements morphological imaging. It is useful:
• To determine whether a focal thyroid nodule or mass is a 'hot nodule' (low incidence of malignancy) or a 'cold nodule' (high incidence of malignancy)
• In hyperthyroidism to distinguish Graves' disease (uniformly increased radionuclide uptake) from toxic adenoma or toxic multinodular goitre (Plummer's disease)

• Postoperatively in patients with thyroid cancer to search for residual local disease and distant metastases
• To identify ectopic thyroid tissue.

Medications such as propylthiouracil and iodine-containing contrast agents may temporarily interfere with the organification of iodine and should be stopped for adequate periods of time before thyroid nuclear scintigraphy.

PET (see Chapter 2)

Lymphoma, primary malignant epithelial tumours and metastatic lymphadenopathy show increased FDG uptake. PET is useful in whole body staging to determine locoregional extent of disease as well as the presence of distant metastasis. FDG-PET is not indicated in the primary diagnosis of thyroid carcinomas but is useful in demonstrating recurrent or metastatic thyroid carcinoma in patients with increasing thyroglobulin levels but negative radio-iodine scans.

CT and MRI

CT and/or MRI is indicated in:
• *Thyroid malignancies:*
  – When the tumour is suspected to have infiltrated into the surrounding structures
  – To demonstrate cervical nodal metastases and pulmonary metastases (CT)
  – For delineating the extent of intrathoracic extension.
• *Salivary glands:*
  – In sialoadenitis to demonstrate presence and extent of complications such as abscess formation (CT)

– Indicated for imaging very large or parotid deep lobe tumours (MRI)
– Tumours arising from the deep spaces such as the parapharyngeal space that displace and/or invade the salivary glands are also better demonstrated on CT and/or MRI
– MRI is unsurpassed in its ability to demonstrate perineural tumour spread, classically by malignant parotid tumour retrogradely along the facial nerve into the otomastoid cavity.

Thyroid

The thyroid is an endocrine organ. Diseases of the thyroid may present as functional disturbance in the form of endocrinopathy (hyperthyroidism or hypothyroidism) or as morphological anomaly in the form of focal (thyroid nodule) or generalized (goitre) glandular enlargement. While the hormonal disturbance can be assessed by biochemical assays, the evaluation of the structural abnormality requires modern imaging techniques that provide high-resolution images of the anatomical alterations.

The term 'goitre' simply means enlargement of the thyroid gland. It may be caused by simple goitre (the most common cause of which is Graves' disease) or the presence of multiple thyroid nodules (multinodular goitre). It should be remembered that the thyroid may contain multiple nodules without being enlarged, in which case the more appropriate term 'multinodular thyroid' should be used.

The aims of imaging of the thyroid gland include:

- To confirm the clinical suspicion of a thyroid lesion and to determine the nature of the lesion if possible
- When goitre is present to see if there is retrosternal or retroclavicular extension and to assess the mass effect on adjacent structures
- To provide precise real-time guidance for FNAC and biopsy
- To follow-up patients after treatment to exclude locoregional recurrence
- To screen patients with increased risk of developing thyroid malignancies (e.g. patients with Hashimoto's thyroiditis).

Imaging is not very accurate in differentiating benign from malignant thyroid nodules and in this respect FNAC is of utmost importance in establishing the diagnosis.

Commonly encountered thyroid pathologies

Multinodular thyroid

This is the most commonly encountered condition of the thyroid (80%), with a predilection for females. Most patients are asymptomatic, but occasionally may present with pressure symptoms from a rapidly enlarging thyroid mass, usually the result of acute haemorrhage within the nodule.

- *US:* hyperplastic nodules are most commonly isoechoic with well-defined margins; cystic components are present in 60% and may be caused by colloid or haemorrhage (Fig. 10.1)
- *NM:* demonstrates multiple hot and cold nodules; toxic nodules will show increased uptake while suppressing the rest of the gland.

Graves' disease (diffuse toxic goitre)

This is the most common cause of hyperthyroidism, with a female predilection. Patients may have associated thyroid ophthalmopathy, and biochemistry demonstrates elevated T3 and T4, suppressed thyroid-stimulating hormone (TSH) and positive anti-TSH receptor antibody.

- *US:* diffusely enlarged gland with heterogeneously hypoechoic, markedly vascular parenchyma
- *NM:* uniformly markedly increased uptake relative to background.

Thyroid malignancy

Papillary carcinoma

This is the most common thyroid malignancy (60–90%), with a female predilection. Risk factors include exposure to external radiation (especially in childhood), excessive iodine intake, autoimmune thyroid disease, genetic syndromes such as Gardner's and Cowden's syndromes.

Lymph node metastases occur in >50% of patients at the time of diagnosis. Distant metastases to lung and bone occur in 5–7% of cases. Prognosis is excellent despite the high incidence of intraglandular and lymph node metastases.

- *US:* papillary carcinomas are usually hypoechoic and ill-defined with irregular margins. Punctate microcalcification is highly specific for papillary tumours (Fig. 10.2). US is valuable in the follow-up of patients who had undergone thyroidectomy for papillary carcinoma.

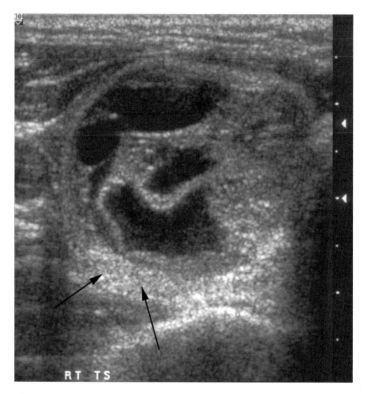

Fig. 10.1 US image of a large complex hyperplastic nodule replacing much of the thyroid right lobe. This lesion contains cystic and solid components. Some normal thyroid tissue is seen posteriorly (black arrows).

Follicular lesion

A follicular carcinoma can only be distinguished from a follicular adenoma by the demonstration of capsular and vascular invasion on histological examination of the entire specimen and the term 'follicular lesion' is thus adopted, which usually implies the need for surgical excision.

Follicular carcinoma accounts for 2–5% of all thyroid malignancies and mostly develops from a pre-existing adenoma. It tends to develop distant

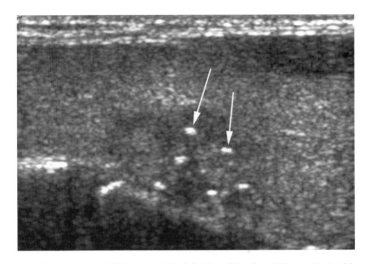

Fig. 10.2 Longitudinal US image of the left lobe of the thyroid in a patient with papillary carcinoma. There is a hypoechoic mass that has poorly defined margins identified and this contains internal fine punctate microcalcifications (white arrows), which represent calcified psammoma bodies.

haematogenous metastases to the lung, liver, bone and brain, with nodal metastases relatively uncommon.
• *US:* follicular carcinomas are largely solid, usually homogeneously hyperechoic lesions and calcification is rare.

Anaplastic carcinoma

This represents 15–20% of all thyroid malignancies with a very aggressive clinical course. There is a predilection for elderly females. It usually presents as a rapidly enlarging thyroid mass causing pressure symptoms. Eighty per cent have a long pre-existing history of goitre.
• *US:* large ill-defined hypoechoic masses replacing the entire lobe are seen.

Adjacent vascular invasion, extracapsular spread and nodal or distant metastases are often present.

Medullary carcinoma

This is uncommon (5% of all thyroid cancers). Medullary carcinoma originates from the calcitonin-producing parafollicular C cells and is associated with multiple endocrine neoplasia (MEN) types 2A and 2B, and C-cell hyperplasia. Nodal metastases are present in 50% at initial presentation, and distant metastases to lung, liver and bone in 15–25%. There is a high recurrence rate, which may be detected by a rising serum calcitonin level.

• *US:* solid hypoechoic nodules, with echogenic foci representing dense amyloid deposits and associated focal calcifications in 80–90%. Multiple or diffuse involvement of both thyroid lobes is almost always seen in the familial form, which has a poor prognosis.

Thyroid lymphoma

Uncommon (1–3% of all thyroid malignancies). Non-Hodgkin's lymphoma is more common in the thyroid and is almost invariably preceded by a history of Hashimoto's thyroiditis. There is a predilection for elderly females. Thyroid lymphoma commonly presents as a rapidly enlarging neck mass.
• *US:* focal lymphomatous nodules and adjacent cervical nodes may show a 'pseudocystic' appearance with posterior acoustic enhancement. Remember thyroid lymphoma does not take up pertechnetate or iodine but is FDG avid.

Thyroiditis

Hashimoto's thyroiditis (autoimmune chronic lymphocytic thyroiditis) is the most common chronic thyroiditis and usually affects middle aged females who present with an often tender goitre and hypothyroidism. Patients are at risk of lymphoma development in particular.

Antibodies against thyroid- and non-thyroid-related proteins serve as the basis of serological diagnosis.
• *US:* may be helpful in gland assessment. An atrophic shrunken thyroid may result.

Salivary glands

Salivary gland diseases usually present clinically as palpable focal or diffuse enlargement. Physical examination often cannot be certain of the exact origin and nature of the palpated lesion and imaging is required to aid in the diagnosis and treatment planning.

Inflammation and neoplasm are the two most common aetiologies of salivary gland diseases. The aim of imaging in the former group is to identify the cause (e.g. ductal obstruction resulting from sialolithiasis) and complications (e.g. abscess formation), while in the latter group imaging is for tumour localization and full extent delineation.

Sialolithiasis

Submandibular stones (80%) are more common than parotid stones because of the higher mucus content of the saliva produced by the submandibular gland. Ninety per cent of submandibular stones are radio–opaque but only 10% of parotid ductal stones are radio–opaque.

Ultrasound is the first-line investigation of choice for the detection of salivary gland stones with high sensitivity, specificity and accuracy (Fig. 10.3). Plain X-rays can be helpful, especially for calculi near the salivary duct meati.

Inflammatory disease

Acute infection

Viral infection (mumps) is a common cause of parotid swelling—imaging is rarely needed. The parotid gland is also most commonly affected by acute

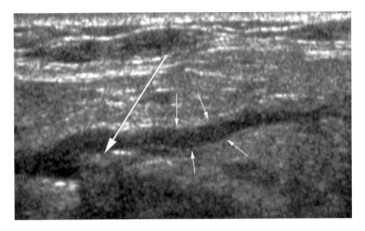

Fig. 10.3 Sonographical features of submandibular sialolithiasis. There is intraglandular ductal dilatation (small white arrows) and intraductal hyperechoic foci are present, consistent with calculi (large white arrow) with associated distal acoustic shadowing.

suppurative sialadenitis, usually secondary to ductal obstruction from sialolithiasis or retrograde entry of oral cavity bacteria. Painful regional adenopathy is often present.

• *US:* the acutely inflamed gland is enlarged with decreased echogenicity. Abscess appears as an ill-defined hypoechoic lesion, sometimes with frank liquefied pus content. Ultrasound-guided aspiration yields specimens for laboratory identification of the culprit organisms and helps in guiding the appropriate antibiotic therapy.

Chronic inflammatory conditions

These are caused by chronic sialolithiasis or other pathology such as Sjögren's syndrome. US is used to confirm or exclude salivary gland involvement in

Sjögren's syndrome and to screen for lymphomatous change in the cervical nodes because patients with Sjögren's syndrome are at increased risk of lymphoma.

Salivary gland neoplasms

US is the initial imaging modality of choice, although US alone is not very accurate in differentiating benign from malignant tumours. Diagnostic accuracy can be further improved by FNAC under US guidance.

Benign neoplasms

Pleomorphic adenoma

Pleomorphic adenoma is the most common salivary gland neoplasm

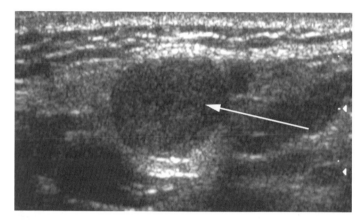

Fig. 10.4 US appearances of a parotid pleomorphic adenoma. There is a rounded, hypoechoic and homogeneous solid mass identified (white arrow) with distal acoustic enhancement.

(60–80%) and 90% arise from the superficial lobe.
• *US:* homogeneous hypoechoic solid masses, rounded or ovoid in shape with well-defined lobulated margins and posterior acoustic enhancement (Fig. 10.4)
• *CT/MR:* can be helpful in delineating large and/or deep lobe lesions or those with atypical US features.

Warthin's tumour

Warthin's tumour (papillary cystadenoma, cystadenolymphoma) accounts for 6–10% of all salivary gland neoplasms and occurs virtually exclusively in the parotid glands. It more commonly affects elderly men; 15–30% of cases are bilateral.
• *US:* typically well-defined hypoechoic lesions with complex internal

heterogeneity comprising of both solid and cystic components.

Malignant neoplasms

Tumours in the sublingual or submandibular glands are more likely to be malignant than tumours in the parotid glands. Imaging features for all malignant tumours are similar and it is not possible to distinguish between the various histopathological subtypes.

Low-grade malignant tumours may appear as well-defined homogeneous lesions mimicking benign tumours; high-grade malignant tumours are more likely to show ill-defined infiltrative margins and heterogeneous internal architecture on all modalities (Fig. 10.5). Cervical and lung metastases may be present.

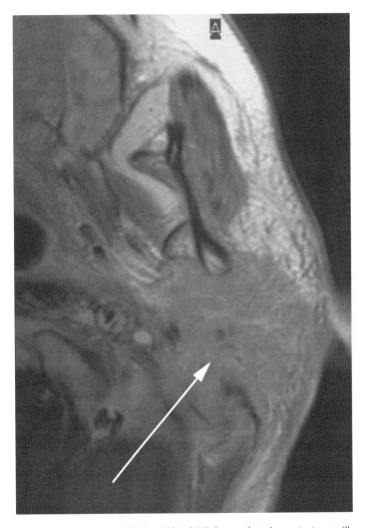

Fig. 10.5 Post-contrast axial T1-weighted MR image that demonstrates an ill-defined enhancing mass replacing the superficial and deep lobes of the left parotid gland (white arrow). Biopsy confirmed this to represent a mucoepidermoid carcinoma.

Mucoepidermoid carcinoma, adenoid cystic carcinoma and acinic cell carcinoma are the main subtypes, with metastases and non-Hodgkin's lymphoma also occasionally identified within the salivary glands.

Cervical lymph nodes

Evaluation of the neck nodal status constitutes an important and integral part of a complete examination for many head and neck diseases. The neck nodal status carries prognostic information and guides the selection of therapy in patients suffering from head and neck cancers. Imaging contributes most significantly to identifying cervical nodal metastatic disease in those patients with no clinically palpable disease (N0). Cervical lymph nodes are also common sites of involvement by lymphoma and tuberculous infection.

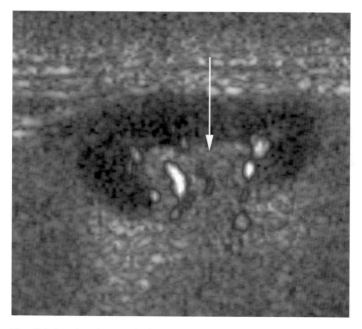

Fig. 10.6 Doppler ultrasound of a normal lymph node. This has an elliptical shape with a central hyperechoic hilum (white arrow) and there is central hilar vascularity.

US

US represents the initial imaging modality of choice for a suspected enlarged cervical node.

Normal cervical nodes appear flat or elliptical, with an echogenic fatty hilum and a hypoechoic cortex (Fig. 10.6). Malignant nodes tend to be more ovoid, hypoechoic and hypervascular, with loss or displacement of the normal fatty hilum (Fig. 10.7). Metastatic cervical lymphadenopathy follows the pattern of lymphatic drainage and tends to be site-specific, which may serve as the hint in localizing unknown primary tumours.

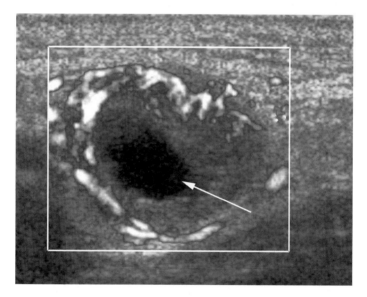

Fig. 10.7 Colour Doppler US of a node involved by metastatic carcinoma. This lesion is rounded and of heterogeneous internal architecture with prominent internal necrosis (white arrow). There is predominantly peripheral and chaotic vascularity consistent with metastatic infiltration.

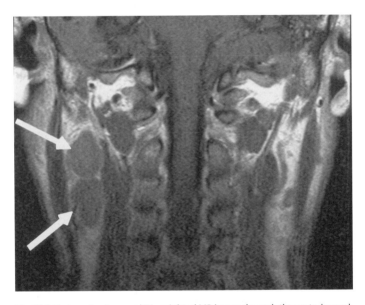

Fig. 10.8 Post-contrast coronal T1-weighted MR image through the posterior neck demonstrating metastatic right-sided cervical adenopathy (white arrows), following the lymphatic drainage from a primary nasopharyngeal carcinoma.

CT and MR

These are used for formal nodal staging in carcinoma and lymphoma (Fig. 10.8). They will not detect metastasis in normal-sized nodes and not all enlarged nodes are malignant. PET may be helpful in some cases.

Further reading

Ahuja AT, Evans R, eds. *Practical Head and Neck Ultrasound*. London: Greenwich Medical Media, 2000.

Chapter 11: **The urogenital tract**

This chapter covers:
Common conditions
• Kidney: renal failure, obstruction, calculus disease, cyst disease, infection, renal cell carcinoma and infection
• Ureter and bladder: calculus, obstruction, tumour
• Prostate: carcinoma
• Testis: tumour, acute scrotum
Common presentations in which imaging can help
• Haematuria: calculus disease, urogenital tract tumour
• Urinary tract infection: calculus disease, obstruction
• Loin pain: tumour, infection, colic from calculus or clot
• Abdominal mass: renal or bladder tumour, renal cyst
• Renal failure: imaging is particularly useful in demonstrating obstruction as a cause, and delineating level and aetiology
• Testicular mass: tumour
• Testicular pain: torsion, tumour, varicocoele, epididymo-orchitis, referred from kidney

Imaging strategy

Note:
That cystoscopy is the primary modality for investigation of the bladder

US

US is the workhorse of uroradiological investigation. It is the primary tool in assessment of renal masses, tumours or cysts and for the symptomatic scrotum. In the assessment of renal failure, US should be performed to exclude a post-renal (obstructive) cause for this presentation. US is often combined with AXR as the initial investigation of haematuria.

AXR

AXR is particularly useful in demonstrating renal tract calcification, whether as calculi or in association with cysts and tumours.

IVU

IVU includes administration of intravenous iodinated contrast (non-ionic) and hence is contraindicated in the presence of renal impairment and iodine allergy. It is still an extremely useful investigation in suspected renal colic, and may be invaluable in the demonstration of urothelial abnormality. IVU may be performed as a second-line investigation of haematuria if US or cystoscopy are unhelpful. Other contrast studies (e.g. cystogram, micturating cystogram, retrograde ureterogram) are usually performed as second-line investigations.

CT

The primary urological function of CT is in the staging and follow-up of primary urogenital tract tumours. CT has a role in further evaluation of renal infection and abscess, and also in the evaluation of complex renal cysts. In some departments, unenhanced CT is used to investigate renal colic, allowing good visualization of ureteric calculi while avoiding iodinated contrast medium.

MRI

This may be helpful in local assessment of bladder or prostatic carcinoma.

NM

NM is not used as a primary imaging modality in renal tract disease.

Renal failure

US is the single most useful investigation for assessment of patients with renal impairment. It can demonstrate:
• Normal kidneys (Fig. 11.1)
• The presence of two kidneys
• Hydronephrosis secondary to mechanical obstruction
• Small shrunken kidneys in chronic renal failure
• Renal or bladder calculi

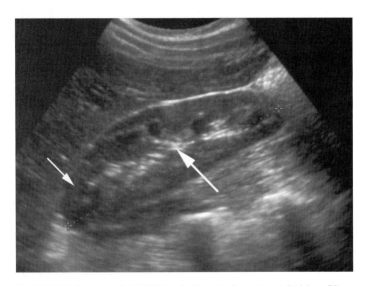

Fig. 11.1 US of a normal right kidney (callipers) adjacent to right lobe of liver. Note normal renal cortex (small white arrow), which appears hypoechoic in relation to hyperechoic renal sinus fat (large white arrow).

- Bladder distension in bladder outflow obstruction.

Further imaging is usually reserved for patients with suspected obstruction.

Urinary tract obstruction

Urinary tract obstruction may be unilateral or bilateral, and can occur at any level from the kidney to the urethra.

Causes include:

- *Kidney:* stone, tumour, blood clot, pelviureteric junction (PUJ) obstruction
- *Ureter:* stone, tumour, stricture, extrinsic compression or invasion (e.g. retroperitoneal fibrosis or tumour)
- *Bladder:* tumour, stone, prostatic hypertrophy
- *Urethra:* stricture, congenital valves.

Acute presentation is often unilateral, with renal colic and pain from the affected flank to the inguinal region. The most common cause is an impacted renal calculus, but impaction of clot or a sloughed papilla can give a similar presentation.

AXR

AXR is used to demonstrate radio-opaque calculi (90% are opaque).

US

US is used to demonstrate hydronephrosis (Fig. 11.2) and calculi. US is

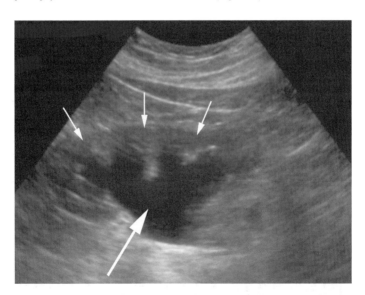

Fig. 11.2 US image of a hydronephrotic kidney. Note the dilatation of the pelvicalyceal system (large white arrow) and thinning of the renal cortex (small white arrows). Cortical thinning suggests chronicity, secondary to prostatic hypertrophy in this case.

accurate in detecting renal or bladder calculi, but ureteric visualization in the retroperitoneum is usually limited.

IVU

IVU will give functional as well as anatomical information. It is frequently the only investigation performed in patients with suspected calculus colic (Fig. 11.3). Classically, the findings on IVU are:
• Increasingly dense nephrogram
• Delayed excretion of contrast to pelvicalyceal system
• Mild to moderate dilatation of collecting system and ureter to the level of obstruction.

US and IVU will both demonstrate dilated collecting systems and will also demonstrate the degree to which renal parenchyma has atrophied (Fig. 11.2). Remember, IVU is contraindicated with renal impairment.

CT

CT is used in some departments in preference to IVU as it allows a quick location of calculus without the need for iodinated contrast. CT is of value in evaluating both the level and often the nature of the obstruction.

Chronic obstruction may be virtually asymptomatic. It may present during investigation for other entities or as a result of a complication such as infection of the obstructed system or deterioration in renal function.

Urinary tract calcification

Urinary calculus

Most commonly formed of oxalate, calcium oxalate or phosphate, uric acid or cystine. A number of conditions predispose:
• Urinary stasis (secondary to obstruction)
• Urinary sepsis
• Metabolic causes (e.g. hyperparathyroidism, hypercalcaemia with hypercalciuria, gout).

Calculi are frequently discovered as an incidental finding. Presenting features include pain, haematuria or evidence of infection.

AXR

Plain film will show many calculi. There is a range of visibility extending from the most obvious staghorn calculus (Fig. 11.4) to radiolucent uric acid calculus. Paradoxically, the latter may often have the more dramatic presentation by causing acute obstruction. FAXR should always be performed prior to a contrast study as valuable information about calculi may be masked by the contrast (Fig. 11.5a,b).

US

US can show calculi within the kidney or occasionally at the vesico-ureteric junction. Demonstration of pelvicalyceal dilatation can be helpful in showing that there is obstruction.

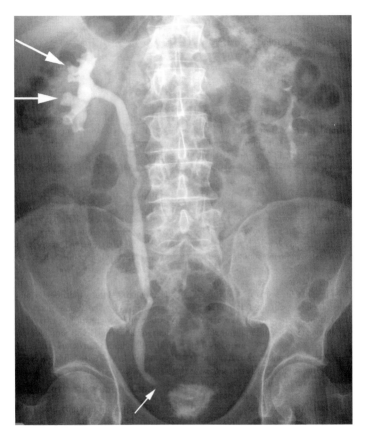

Fig. 11.3 A post-micturition film performed in an IVU series in a patient with right renal colic. This demonstrates mild right-sided pelvicalyceal dilatation with calyceal clubbing (large white arrows) and dilatation of the right ureter also down to the level of the vesico-ureteric junction (small white arrow). This was secondary to a radiolucent calculus.

IVU

IVU allows delineation of renal tract anatomy and its relationship to calculi seen on plain film. Delayed excretion into a dilated pelvicalyceal system or ureter indicates the presence of obstruction, and with time its level.

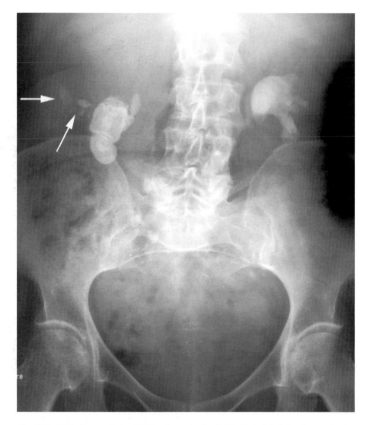

Fig. 11.4 AXR demonstrates bilateral renal calculi. The left-sided staghorn calculus has a configuration similar to the pelvicalyceal system that it fills. On the right side there is a large calculus lying in the renal pelvis and upper right ureter, with smaller calculi seen in the lower pole of the right kidney (arrows).

CT

CT may be offered in some departments in place of IVU as it allows demonstration of calculus without the need for contrast agents.

CT will show high density of calculus, thus allowing distinction from urothelial tumour (where confusion could occur with radiolucent calculus on IVU).

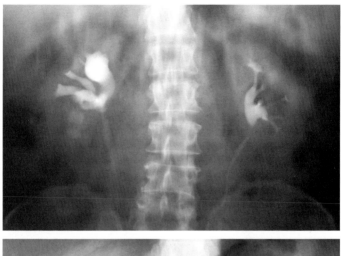

a

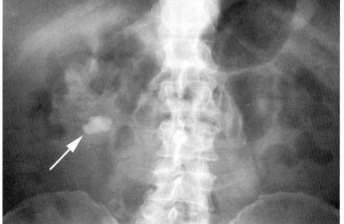

b

Fig. 11.5 (a) An image from IVU series post-contrast administration. This demonstrates right-sided pelvicalyceal dilatation although no definite cause is seen. (b) A control pre-injection radiograph in the same patient as (a) confirms the presence of a large calculus at the pelviureteric junction that is causing obstruction (arrow). This was obscured on post-contrast images.

Nephrocalcinosis

Cortical nephrocalcinosis

This is visible on AXR as calcification predominantly in the renal cortex. Causes are acute cortical necrosis, chronic glomerulonephritis and oxalosis.

Medullary nephrocalcinosis

This appears as grouped medullary rounded and linear calcifications on AXR (Fig. 11.6). Causes are hyperparathyroidism, renal tubular acidosis, medullary sponge kidney (Fig. 11.6) and hyperoxaluria.

Focal calcification

Calcification may occur in a renal mass and may be malignant in 75% of cases. Causes include:

- Tumour
- Infection: commonly tuberculous or xanthogranulomatous pyelonephritis
- Cysts: secondary to haemorrhage or previous infection.
- Vascular.

Renal cyst disease

Simple cyst

This represents the most common renal mass lesion representing approximately 60% of the total. The incidence of such cysts increases with increasing age. These lesions are, by definition, simple with a thin wall and containing only serous fluid. Simple cysts are most commonly found incidentally while investigating other conditions. Occasionally, the cyst may become so large as to cause abdominal discomfort and a palpable

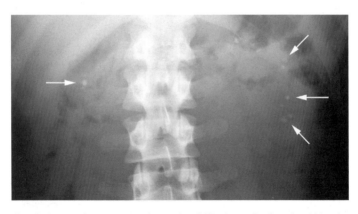

Fig. 11.6 AXR demonstrates clustered calcifications distributed within the medullary regions of the kidneys bilaterally (arrows) in a patient with medullary sponge kidney. In this condition there is cystic dilatation of the papillary and medullary portions of the collecting ducts and calcifications may form within them.

mass. These cysts may also present through complicating episodes of haemorrhage or infection and, occasionally, a large cyst may cause obstruction if it lies adjacent to the upper ureter and renal pelvis.

US

Simple cysts are frequently detected incidentally using US. US is also the modality of choice for cyst characterization (Fig. 11.7). Haemorrhage and/or infection may cause debris in cysts, which can mimic tumour and follow-up is needed. If the cyst is demonstrated on US to be simple (thin-walled) with homogeneous fluid content and well demarcated from the rest of the kidney then no further investigation is required.

IVU

A simple cyst, if large enough, may be demonstrated as a mass lesion. Its

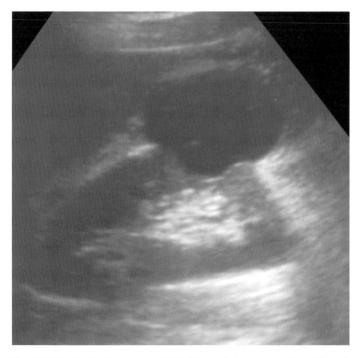

Fig. 11.7 US of a simple renal cyst. This is thin-walled and anechoic and there is distal acoustic enhancement.

low density may give a clue as to its nature.

CT and MR

CT and/or MR will clearly demonstrate simple cysts, which are often an incidental finding on abdominal examinations, and may be used to further evaluate or follow-up complex cysts.

Adult polycystic disease

There is autosomal dominant inheritance and therefore there is likely to be a strong family history. Cysts of varying sizes are first present in early adulthood and progress in those severely affected to give two large kidneys (which are often palpable) that are largely cystic, eventually leading to renal failure.

US is the best tool for initial assessment (Fig. 11.8) and monitoring progress, but CT and MRI may be useful in distinguishing haemorrhagic or infected cysts from malignancy.

Urinary tract infection

Pyelonephritis

Acute pyelonephritis refers to acute upper urinary tract infection, most often by pathogenic coliform bacteria that have entered the lower urinary tract via the urethra. As a result of longer urethra and antibacterial properties of prostatic

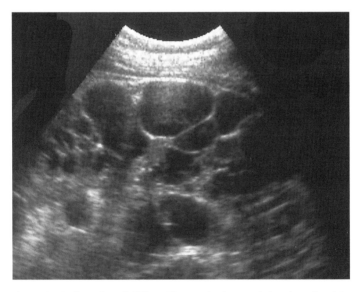

Fig. 11.8 US of a polycystic kidney. The renal substance is largely replaced by multiple cysts of varying sizes and the kidney is grossly enlarged.

secretions, males are far less frequently affected than females.

Presentation is with:
• Fever
• Frequency
• Flank pain
• Dysuria
• Bacteria and pus cells in urine.

Imaging

Imaging is not required for uncomplicated cases. US and AXR may provide further information when patient has:
• Diabetes
• Previous urinary calculi
• Atypical organism
• Poor response to treatment
• Frequent recurrences.

Renal abscess

Diabetics are predisposed. Sepsis arises from ascending, usually Gram negative, organisms in 80% of cases, with haematogenous spread in 20%.

US

US will show a hypoechoic mass progressing to an anechoic mass in later stages, as a result of liquefaction, with an irregular margin to the lesion.

CT

CT shows focal necrotic mass with enhancement of thickened margins. It may be hard to differentiate from tumour.

Emphysematous pyelonephritis

Emphysematous pyelonephritis is a renal infection with gas-forming organisms, with a 40–50% mortality. It occurs in predisposed patients:
• Immunocompromised, particularly diabetics.
• Those with obstructed kidney. Gas in the renal interstitial and perirenal tissues may be seen on AXR (Fig. 11.9) and CT.

Renal cell carcinoma

This tumour represents 80–90% of all renal malignancy, with peak prevalence seen in the sixth decade. Renal cell carcinoma is bilateral in 2% of patients. Bilateral and multicentric tumours are common in patients with von Hippel–Lindau syndrome.

Presentation is with:
• Often an incidental CT or US finding during the investigation of other symptoms
• *Local symptoms:* haematuria, pain, mass
• *General:* weight loss, fever, varicocoele (sudden appearance on left because of compression of left gonadal vein), anaemia, hypercalcaemia
• *Metastases* (25% at presentation): bone pain, cough, haemoptysis.

AXR

AXR may show:
• Calcification of renal mass
• Bulge in renal contour
• Pulmonary metastases
• Bony metastases (may be expansile).

US

US of renal cell carcinoma can have

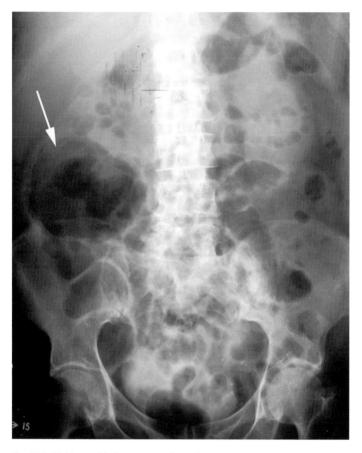

Fig. 11.9 AXR in an elderly patient with emphysematous pyelonephritis. Note the presence of air within the right renal substance (arrow).

variable appearances. Necrosis will give areas of low echogenicity in the centre of many tumours, particularly the larger ones. US is particularly helpful in demonstrating extension of tumour to the inferior vena cava (Fig. 11.10), which, if extensive, will significantly affect treatment planning.

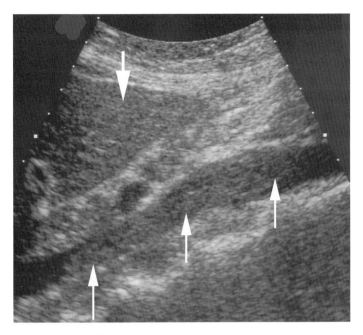

Fig. 11.10 Sagittal US of the inferior vena cava in a patient with renal cell carcinoma, demonstrating hypoechoic tumour thrombus (white arrows) within the inferior vena cava. Note normal liver (white arrow head).

CT

This is the most sensitive technique for further characterization of renal masses (Fig. 11.11) but also an essential tool in local staging and demonstration of lymph node spread. Evidence of renal vein extension may also be shown.

MRI

MRI has no definite role at present but may be helpful in imaging patients with allergy to iodinated contrast.

IVU

IVU is of limited use as it demonstrates features of mass lesion but does not distinguish it from renal cyst.

Angiography

Angiography is no longer part of diagnostic imaging strategy but may be used as part of tumour embolization for palliation in those unsuitable for curative surgery.

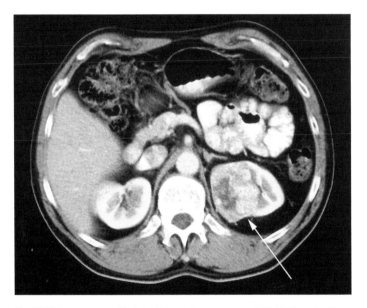

Fig. 11.11 Post-contrast CT of the kidneys demonstrates a left-sided renal cell carcinoma. There is a mixed attenuation mass arising medially from the left kidney (arrow). Note central low attenuation consistent with necrosis.

Urothelial tumours

These tumours arise from the lining epithelium anywhere in the renal tract. Eighty per cent are transitional cell carcinomas (TCCs) and 15% are squamous cell carcinomas. They arise most commonly in the bladder and least frequently in the ureter.

TCC is associated with:
- Exposure to aniline dyes
- Tobacco
- Cyclophosphamide therapy
- Pelvic radiation.

Males are more commonly affected than females in a ratio of 3 : 1.

Painless haematuria is the most common presenting feature (in up to 90% of cases). This finding may be associated with irritative symptoms of dysuria, urgency and frequency. Patients may also present with obstruction and frequency without haematuria.

Most of these tumours arise in the bladder and so investigation and diagnosis is largely the preserve of the cystoscopist. Investigation is designed around the causes of haematuria.

AXR

Calcification may occasionally be demonstrable encrusted onto the surface of the tumour or punctate within the lesion. Radio–opaque calculi will also be demonstrated by this examination.

US

US is of value in detecting soft-tissue tumours of the upper urinary tract and will also demonstrate evidence of obstruction by tumour in the lower urinary tract. Bladder tumour may also be demonstrated by US.

IVU

If the cause for haematuria remains elusive, IVU will allow visualization of the pelvicalyceal systems and ureters in the search for filling defects suggestive of TCC. Blood clots, however, can give similar appearances.

Retrograde pyelogram

This allows visualization of the pelvicalyceal systems and ureters, as with the IVU, but is performed by instilling iodinated contrast via ureteric catheters placed cystoscopically (Fig. 11.12). During fluoroscopy there is greater control, allowing for more detailed examination which may be targeted at areas of uncertainty on the IVU. Brush biopsy of suspicious filling defects should be possible if the ureteric catheter is left in place.

CT

CT is invaluable as a tool for the staging of urothelial tumours, allowing assessment of local and distant metastatic spread. CT can be used to guide biopsy of enlarged lymph nodes in order to confirm tumour involvement.

MRI

MRI can provide improved detail of local invasion, particularly in respect of the depth of muscle invasion by bladder tumour. Often, local staging will be based on clinical or pathological grounds alone.

Squamous cell carcinoma

Squamous cell carcinoma is rare but often found in association with chronic irritation of the epithelium, particularly from calculi but also from schistosomiasis. It has a poor prognosis as a result of early metastases.

Other causes

Other causes of a mass in the pelvicalyceal system are as follows:
• Uric acid calculi (radiolucent)
• Vascular impressions
• Tuberculosis
• Pyeloureteritis cystica
• Papillary necrosis (sloughed papilla)
• Renal cell carcinoma extending into pelvicalyceal system
• Metastases (e.g. melanoma).

Prostatic carcinoma

This is the most common of all urinary tract cancers, but frequently remains latent and undiscovered. The tumour arises in the peripheral zone (70%)

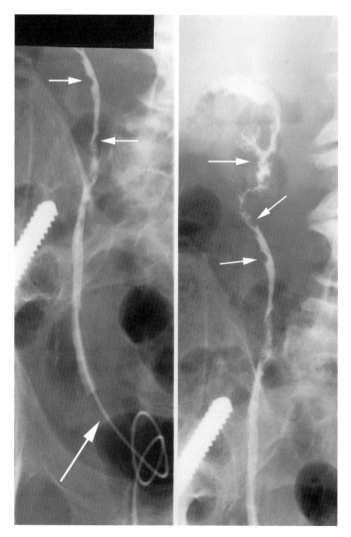

Fig. 11.12 Films from a right retrograde pyelogram study. Contrast has been injected into a catheter lying in the right ureter (large white arrow) introduced cystoscopically. Note extensive irregular filling defects (small white arrows) within the pelvicalyceal system and ureter consistent with diffuse transitional cell carcinoma.

and almost all are adenocarcinoma (>95%).

Presentation is with:

- Prostatism
- Haematuria
- Bone pain from metastasis or pathological fracture
- Renal failure secondary to obstruction by local infiltration of distal ureters.

The crucial issue is in determining suitability for radical treatment. At present, this is done mainly on clinical, biochemical and histological grounds.

Radiography

X-rays demonstrate the sclerotic lesions that are characteristic of prostate secondaries in bone (Fig. 11.13) and also pathological fractures.

US

Transabdominal and transrectal US can show prostate carcinoma as a hypoechoic lesion, although a variety of appearances are described. A significant number of cancers cannot be demonstrated by US. US is a good tool for directing transrectal biopsy and will demonstrate upper tract obstruction.

CT

CT demonstrates gross local invasion of adjacent structures and also evidence of

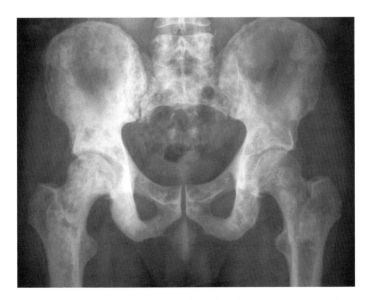

Fig. 11.13 Pelvic radiograph in a patient with metastatic prostate carcinoma. There are multiple sclerotic metastases present.

distant spread such as lymph node enlargement. However, it cannot allow accurate enough local staging to determine suitability for radical treatment.

MRI

MRI gives better detail of local anatomy and therefore better local staging. There is controversy at present whether local staging is accurate enough to allow decisions to be made for or against radical treatment.

NM

If prostate-specific antigen (PSA) is significantly raised then isotope bone scan allows a sensitive one-stop survey of the entire skeleton for bony deposits. If clinical suspicion for a targeted area remains high in the face of negative bone scan, then MR is of value.

The testis

Testicular tumour

This is the most common tumour in males between 25 and 35 years of age. Seminoma and teratoma are the most common subtypes. Patients tend to present with painless enlargement of a testis. Pain and/or hydrocoele may occur and occasionally patients present with symptoms of metastatic disease.

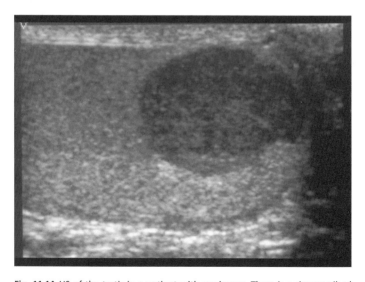

Fig. 11.14 US of the testis in a patient with seminoma. There is a circumscribed hypoechoic mass in the lower pole of the testicle that was confirmed as a seminoma.

US

US is the required initial investigation. It is extremely sensitive in the detection and characterization of testicular masses and also for differentiating intra- and extratesticular lesions. The US features of testicular tumours vary: seminoma frequently appears hypoechoic and solid (Fig. 11.14), with teratoma containing solid, cystic and calcific components.

Recently, the phenomenon of testicular microlithiasis has been revealed with high-resolution US equipment. This represents tiny foci of microcalcification in testicular tubules (Fig. 11.15) and is thought to be associated with the development of malignant tumour, especially seminoma.

CT

CT is used to stage malignant testicular tumours, demonstrating para-aortic lymphadenopathy and hepatic or pulmonary lesions. CT is used in combination with tumour markers to monitor response to treatment.

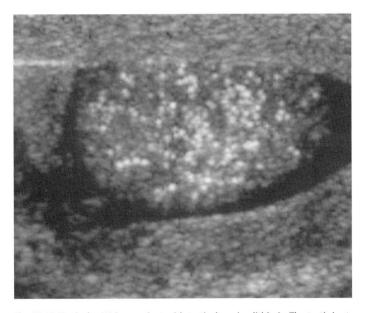

Fig. 11.15 Testicular US in a patient with testicular microlithiasis. The testis is atrophic, which may be related to previous inflammation, and in addition there are multiple hyperechoic flecks seen throughout the testicular parenchyma. Such patients need clinical and sonographic follow-up to exclude tumour development.

The acute scrotum

Epididymo-orchitis

US is accurate in diagnosing acute scrotal inflammation and is helpful if abscess formation is suspected.

Torsion

Torsion may have complex and confus-ing appearances on US so if there is clinical concern about possible torsion, the scrotum should always be surgically explored.

Further reading

Dahnert W, ed. *Radiology Review Manual*, 5th edn. Philadelphia: Lippincott Williams & Wilkins, 2003.

Chapter 12: **Central nervous system**

This chapter covers:
Common conditions involving the brain and spine
- **Trauma**
- **Cerebrovascular disease**
- **Subarachnoid haemorrhage**
- **Infection**
- **Tumours**
- **Multiple sclerosis**
- **Cord compression**

Common presentations in which imaging can help
- **Collapse: stroke, haemorrhage, trauma**
- **Headache: haemorrhage, tumour, infection**
- **Fit: tumour, infection, stroke, haemorrhage**
- **Funny turn: transient ischaemic attack, tumour**
- **Altered conscious level: trauma, infection, stroke, haemorrhage**

Imaging strategy

Most patients with neurological symptoms and signs require cerebral imaging as part of their management, usually CT or MRI, or both. Plain X-rays rarely supply any additional information.

In the acute setting, usually following trauma or collapse, the patient must be resuscitated and stabilized first, before any imaging is considered. If the patient is agitated or confused, the anaesthetist must be contacted early to intubate or sedate the patient and communication with the radiologist is advised.

The decision as to which modality to use is dependent on a number of factors. Some of the advantages and disadvantages of CT and MRI are as follow.

Advantages of CT

- Fast
- Usually available out of normal working hours
- Sensitive for detection of intracranial blood, and excellent bone detail.

Disadvantages of CT

- Involves ionizing radiation
- Views of the posterior fossa are degraded by artefact from skull base.

Advantages of MRI

- Multiplanar imaging ideal for accurate localization of a lesion
- Wide coverage (e.g. whole spine can be imaged to identify level of cord compression)
- No ionizing radiation
- Very sensitive in detection of small lesions and involvement of the meninges, cranial nerves and posterior fossa.

Disadvantages of MRI

- Slow (relatively)
- Images degraded by slight movement

• Unsuitable for patients with pacemakers, recent surgery or claustrophobia (see Chapter 2)
• Usually not available out of normal working hours
• Poor bony detail
• Special equipment necessary for patient ventilation and monitoring.

Good communication is essential. An accurate neurological assessment can assist greatly in the selection of the most appropriate imaging modality to make a diagnosis. Similarly, the results may require urgent action and the requesting clinician must be readily available to receive and act on the imaging findings.

Trauma

Patients with major trauma often need resuscitation and stabilization before imaging. If there are multiple sites of injury, the full extent of imaging required should be agreed before commencement. About one-third of patients with significant brain injury do not have a skull fracture, and the presence of a fracture does not necessarily indicate an associated brain injury. Traditionally, UK practice has relied heavily on skull radiography, but this should now largely be reserved for when CT is not available or for suspected non-accidental injury. CT is advised in those patients where brain injury is suspected clinically.

CT

When intracranial haematoma or brain injury is suspected, CT is the best initial imaging modality. MRI may be appropriate if the patient's clinical and CT

appearances do not correlate and also to identify small contusions and subtle abnormalities in the brainstem or posterior fossa. Patients who are fully orientated and have no history of loss of consciousness do not require brain imaging.

National Institute for Clinical Excellence (NICE) guidelines for imaging adults with serious head injury are as follow:
• Glasgow coma score (GCS) < 13
• Suspected open or depressed skull fracture
• Any sign of basal skull fracture (e.g. cerebrospinal fluid [CSF] otorrhoea, racoon eyes, Battle's sign)
• Repeated vomiting
• Post-traumatic seizure
• Focal neurological deficit
• Coagulopathy.
Even if CT is normal, these patients usually require admission and observation.

Extradural haematoma

Extradural haematomas (EDHs) are most common in the fronto-parietal region resulting from direct injury to the middle meningeal artery, but can occur in the posterior fossa when the accumulation of blood occurs between the skull and the dura.

On CT, an EDH typically appears as a biconvex high-density lesion deep to the skull vault that is often fractured. There is usually considerable cerebral mass effect (Figs 12.1 & 12.2).

Patients with EDHs are often lucid for several hours after the trauma, but may show a rapid decline in their level of consciousness as the haematoma continues to enlarge, causing mass effect and cerebral herniation.

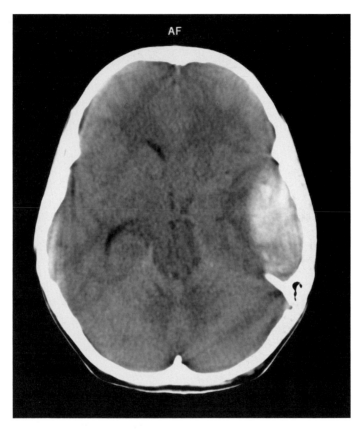

Fig. 12.1 CT shows a left-sided extradural haematoma. Note the biconvex shape, mass effect and effacement of the temporal and anterior horns of the left lateral ventricle.

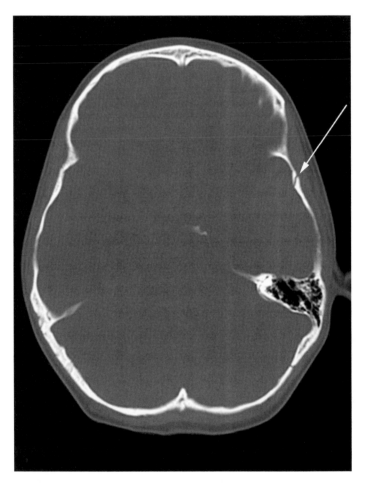

Fig. 12.2 CT using a bone window setting in the same patient as Fig. 12.1 demonstrates the left temporal bone fracture (arrow).

Subdural haematoma

There is usually a history of head trauma but this may be relatively minor, especially in elderly or alcoholic patients. Most patients with a subdural haematoma (SDH) have a neurological deficit, personality change or altered consciousness level. The accumulation of blood in SDH occurs between the dura and arachnoid mater and is caused by the tearing of bridging veins.

An acute SDH is shown as a crescentic rather than biconcave area of increased density on CT, most commonly in the parietal region. The density of the haematoma on CT imaging decreases with time. After the initial bleed, blood appears hyperdense, becoming the same density (isodense) as adjacent brain after 2 weeks, and after 3 weeks it is of lower density than brain. A chronic SDH is often the same density as CSF (Fig. 12.3).

Acute-on-chronic SDHs are not uncommon in alcoholics and show blood of different densities according to age (Fig. 12.3).

Cerebrovascular disease

Cerebral infarction

Cerebrovascular accident (CVA) or stroke are terms given to an underlying cerebrovascular disorder usually caused by atherosclerosis, thrombosis, embolism, hypoperfusion, vasculitis or venous stasis. CT is usually used in the initial assessment to identify cerebral haemorrhage or underlying vascular malformations and tumours that may mimic stroke symptoms. If an infarct (and no bleed) is present, the patient is usually commenced on aspirin or another form of anticoagulation.

An abnormality is usually seen on CT after 24 hours following onset of symptoms in patients with cerebral infarcts. These are usually areas of low density affecting both white and grey matter in a vascular distribution (Fig. 12.4). CT scans performed earlier are often normal. MRI is more sensitive than CT at early infarct detection, but these patients are usually agitated and are unable to lie still enough in the acute setting. MRI is useful for identifying brainstem and posterior fossa infarcts that may not be well demonstrated on CT.

Twenty to 25% of large infarcts become haemorrhagic infarcts, usually between 24–48 hours after the ischaemic event and these show areas of increased density within the area of infarction.

Transient ischaemic attack

Patients with transient ischaemic attacks (TIAs; neurological symptoms or signs resolved in <24 hours), or those who have made good neurological improvement following a cerebral infarction, should also undergo a carotid duplex ultrasound scan if they are considered suitable candidates for surgical treatment of their arteries (e.g. carotid endarterectomy). Although there is no age limit, the risks of surgery in patients older than 85 years often exceed benefit. The duplex scan identifies plaques within the internal and common carotid arteries causing areas of stenosis or narrowing. At the site of stenosis, the velocity of the blood flow in the vessel increases in proportion to the degree of narrowing and the amount of stenosis can be calculated (Figs 12.5 & 12.6).

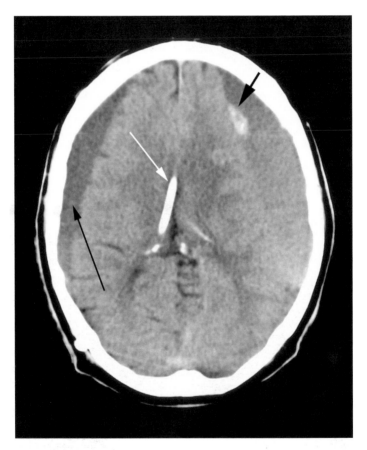

Fig. 12.3 CT of a patient with a right-sided intraventricular shunt (white arrow).
Note the low-density right-sided chronic SDH (long black arrow) and the acute on
chronic left-sided SDH. This is shown as a mixed increased and low-density area
suggesting an acute bleed into an existing chronic SDH. A focus of acute haemorrhage is present (small black arrow).

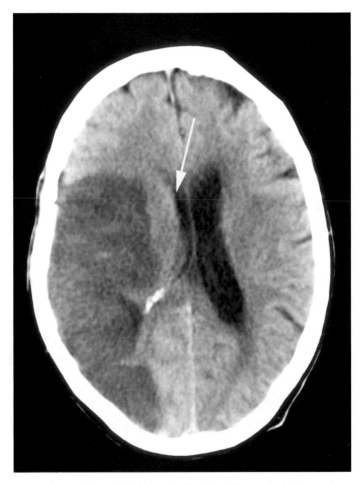

Fig. 12.4 CT scan shows a large infarct in the right middle cerebral artery territory. This is a low-density defect involving both white and grey matter. There is associated mass effect with the right lateral ventricle partially effaced (arrow) and there is minor mid line shift to the left.

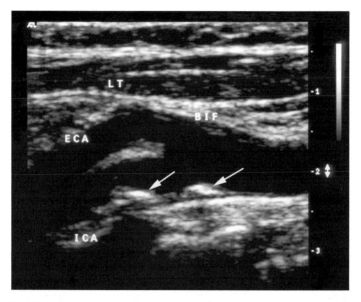

Fig. 12.5 Left carotid artery US scan showing large atherosclerotic plaques (arrows) at the origin of the internal carotid artery (ICA). The external carotid artery (ECA) and bifurcation (BIF) are also annotated.

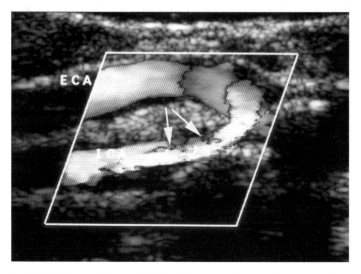

Fig. 12.6 Colour duplex carotid US in the same patient as Fig. 12.5 confirms significant ICA narrowing secondary to the plaque with flow turbulence (arrows).

Intracerebral haematoma

Hypertensive haemorrhage is the most common cause of spontaneous intracerebral haematoma. Patients commonly present with similar symptoms and signs to a cerebral infarct, with sudden-onset neurological deficit, possibly with altered conscious level, depend-ing upon the size and amount of mass effect of the bleed. Patients are frequently sedation or confused and may require sedation or intubation prior to imaging.

Most intracerebral haemorrhages occur within the cerebral hemispheres, especially within the basal ganglia, but 20% occur in the brainstem or cerebellum. CT demonstrates a well-defined area of high density (Fig. 12.7).

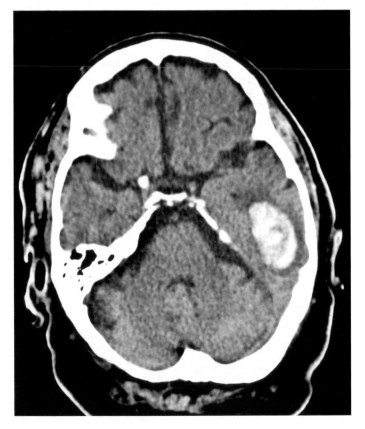

Fig. 12.7 Unenhanced CT scan demonstrates an acute left temporal lobe haematoma.

Cerebellar haematomas can be amenable to neurosurgical evacuation so urgent consultation with a neurosurgeon may be appropriate.

Subarachnoid haemorrhage

Patients with subarachnoid haemorrhage (SAH) typically present with severe sudden-onset headache, frequently occipital. Ninety per cent of non-traumatic SAHs are caused by ruptured berry aneurysms. In order of frequency, these arise from the:

- Posterior communicating artery
- Anterior communicating artery
- Middle cerebral artery
- Internal carotid artery
- Tip of the basilar artery.

Other causes include arteriovenous (AV) malformations, hypertensive haemorrhage, anticoagulation therapy and trauma.

CT

CT is indicated, particularly if the patient has a deteriorating or fluctuating consciousness level or a neurological deficit. Patients may require sedation or intubation if they are confused or agitated prior to imaging.

CT will demonstrate a SAH in approximately 80% of cases. The normal low-density CSF is replaced by high-density blood in the basal cisterns and/or sulci (Fig. 12.8).

Patients with normal CT scans and no clinical signs of raised intracranial pressure should undergo lumbar puncture to demonstrate xanthochromia and make the diagnosis of SAH.

Hydrocephalus that is acute obstructive (occurring within 1 week) or delayed communicating (occurring after 1 week), cerebral vasospasm and infarction, and transtentorial herniation are recognized complications.

Urgent contact with a neurosurgical centre is advised once the diagnosis is made. The patient may undergo cerebral angiography to identify the cause, embolization or surgical clipping of the aneurysm and intraventricular shunt insertion if there is hydrocephalus.

MRA

MRA may sometimes be useful in demonstrating the aneurysm (Fig. 12.9); however, small aneurysms are not always detected.

Cerebral infection

Meningitis

Patients with suspected meningitis present acutely, are usually unwell, febrile and have signs of meningism such as neck stiffness and photophobia. If a patient has the following clinical signs, CT is indicated to exclude the presence of a cerebral abscess:

- Altered or fluctuating consciousness level or mental state
- Seizures
- Papilloedema
- Focal neurological deficit.

These patients are usually extremely unwell and may be agitated, often requiring sedation or intubation prior to the CT scan. Early communication with a senior colleague and anaesthetist is advised.

A normal CT scan does not exclude the presence of raised intracranial pressure as this can be present in patients who have a normal CT.

Patients with acute onset of symp-

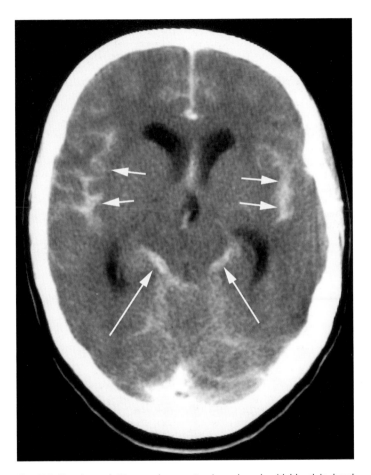

Fig. 12.8 Unenhanced CT scan shows extensive subarachnoid blood in basal cisterns (long arrows), the sylvian fissures (short arrows) and within sulci.

toms and signs of raised intracranial pressure should not undergo lumbar puncture, even in the event of having a normal CT scan.

A CT scan is not indicated for patients with suspected meningitis with no clinical signs of raised intracranial pressure, prior to lumbar puncture.

Cerebral abscess

These are usually caused by pyogenic

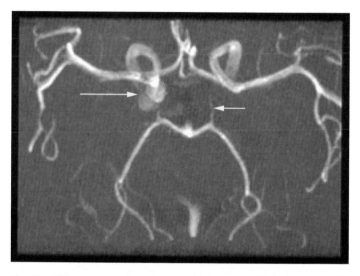

Fig. 12.9 MRA shows a posterior view of the circle of Willis with an aneurysm arising from the right posterior communicating artery (long white arrow). Note normal left posterior communicating artery (short white arrow).

bacteria that reach the brain by direct spread from an open skull fracture or surgery; from localized infection such as meningitis, mastoiditis or sinusitis; or from a distant focus such as bacterial endocarditis or sepsis.

In the emergency setting, CT is usually the investigation of choice. These patients are usually extremely unwell and may be agitated, requiring sedation or intubation prior to the CT scan. Early communication with a senior colleague, an anaesthetist and a radiologist is advised.

CT

On CT, a cerebral abscess is usually an area of low density in the affected white matter, with surrounding low-density oedema and mass effect. When intravenous contrast is administered, there is usually peripheral or ring enhancement (Fig. 12.10). There may be fluid and bone destruction in adjacent sinuses or mastoid air cells. The main radiological differential diagnosis includes primary or secondary cerebral tumour.

MRI

MRI with gadolinium enhancement is more sensitive for early detection of cerebral infection and meningeal involvement; however, the patient needs to be able to lie completely still in order to obtain images of diagnostic quality.

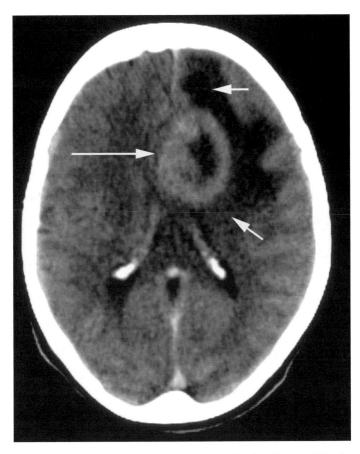

Fig. 12.10 Post-contrast CT scan showing a ring-enhancing abscess within the left fronto-parietal region (long white arrow). Note the large amount of surrounding low-density oedema (small white arrows). The differential diagnosis includes a primary tumour or metastasis.

Cerebral tumours

Cerebral tumours are more common in adults, with a peak incidence at 55–65 years. Patients usually present with focal neurological deficit, personality change or seizures. They may be agitated or confused at presentation.

The most common tumours, in order of their incidence, are:

- Gliomas
- Metastases
- Meningiomas.

Posterior fossa tumours are more common in children than adults. Gliomas may have similar imaging char-acteristics to cerebral abscesses and the diagnosis is often dependent on the clinical findings. The level of contrast enhancement on CT and MRI correlates with the grade of tumour (Fig. 12.11).

Metastases represent approximately 20% of all intracranial tumours, and up to 85% of cases demonstrate more than

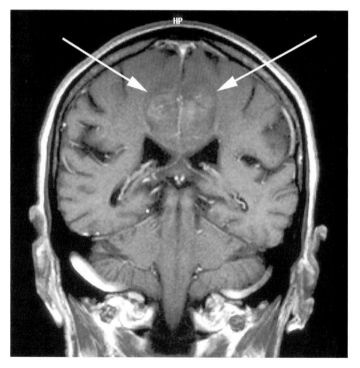

Fig. 12.11 Coronal post-contrast T1-weighted image through the bodies of the lateral ventricles in a patient with a glioma. There is an ill-defined mass crossing the mid line (long arrows), which has some patchy internal enhancement. The main differential diagnosis for lesions that involve the corpus callosum and cross the mid line is glioma or lymphoma.

one lesion. The primary site is most commonly lung, and patients with suspected metastatic disease should have a CXR. Other primary sites include breast, genitourinary and gastrointestinal tracts, thyroid and melanoma. Metastases usually demonstrate contrast enhancement on CT (Fig. 12.12) and MRI. MRI is more sensitive for lesion detection than CT and its multiplanar capability is useful for localizing lesions for biopsy.

Multiple sclerosis

Multiple sclerosis (MS) is a relapsing/remitting demyelinating disorder. Patients present with a spectrum of symptoms, which can be mild such as numbness in hands or feet, or reduced vision, or severe such as hemiplegia or paraplegia. It is more common in women, with 95% of cases occurring between 18 and 50 years.

MRI is the most accurate imaging modality for patients with suspected MS, with a sensitivity of 85%.

MS plaques typically have an oval shape and are bright or high signal on T2-weighted images (Fig. 12.13). They most characteristically occur in the white matter around the ventricles but can also occur in the brainstem, posterior fossa and spinal cord.

The MRI findings are suggestive of MS when three or more lesions >5mm are present in a periventricular location.

As MS is a clinical diagnosis, the appearances are suggestive but not diagnostic of the disease. There are several other causes of white matter disease, such as ischaemia, infection and vasculitic disorders, and so the clinical history is extremely important.

Cord compression

Metastatic disease involving the spine causes neurological deficit in up to 10% of cancer patients. If this results in cord compression, there is a dramatic reduction in the patient's quality of life and life expectancy.

Most spinal metastases occur by haematogenous spread from carcinoma of the:
• Breast
• Lung
• Prostate
• Kidney
• Thyroid.
Spine involvement also occurs with myeloma, lymphoma and leukaemia. Cord compression can also occur with disc prolapse and infection. An urgent MRI scan is indicated if a patient has signs and symptoms of cord compression:
• Reduction or loss of motor function (often lower limb—cauda equina syndrome)
• Reduction or loss of sensation (a sensory level may be demonstrated)
• Bladder dysfunction
• Loss of anal tone.
Discussion with senior colleagues is advised to obtain an urgent MRI scan. This may not be available out of normal working hours and arrangements may be needed to transfer the patient for imaging and treatment. Urgent treatment usually involves radiotherapy or decompressive surgery and this has been shown to significantly reduce morbidity. Be available for imaging results.

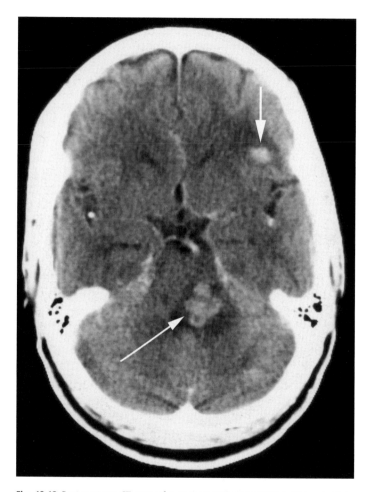

Fig. 12.12 Post-contrast CT scan of a patient with metastatic melanoma. Note the enhancing lesions within the left frontal lobe and the left middle cerebellar peduncle (arrows) and associated low attenuation oedema.

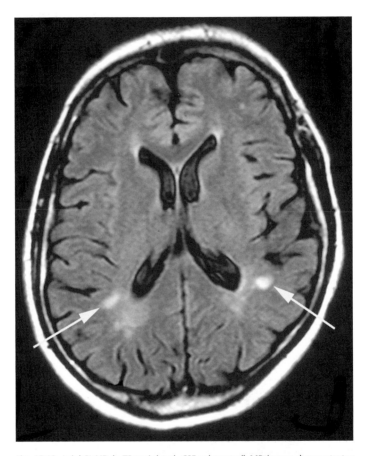

Fig. 12.13 Axial FLAIR (a T2-weighted, CSF subtracted) MR image demonstrates multiple high-signal periventricular lesions (arrows) suggestive of demyelination. FLAIR is a MR sequence sensitive in the detection of MS plaques.

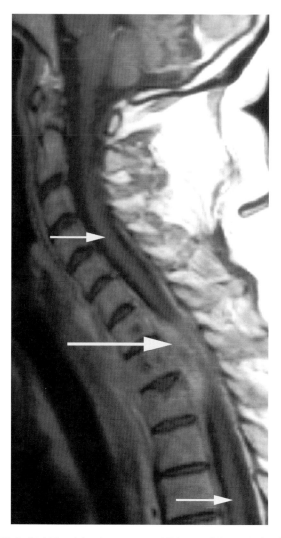

Fig. 12.14 Sagittal T1-weighted post-contrast MR image of the cervical and upper thoracic spine in a patient with known metastatic breast cancer. There is a large plaque of extradural metastatic tumour at the T1/T2 level (large white arrow), which significantly reduces the calibre of the spinal canal and compresses the cord. Note normal cord above and below the level of compression (small white arrows).

MRI

MRI clearly defines the level of abnormality (there may be several) necessary for treatment and is able to demonstrate whether the cord or exiting nerve roots are involved (Fig. 12.14).

Other forms of imaging such as plain radiographs, CT or radioisotope bone scans are far less sensitive and specific.

Further reading

Orrison WW, ed. *Neuroimaging*. Philadelphia: Saunders, 2000.

Index

Note: page numbers in *italics* refer to figures and boxes, those in **bold** refer to tables.

214